# ATLAS OF AVIAN NECROPSY

For this English edition:

Atlas of avian necropsy

Plaza Antonio Beltrán Martínez nº 1, planta 8 - letra I
(Centro empresarial El Trovador)
50002 Zaragoza - Spain

This book has been published originally in Spanish under the title:
*Atlas de la necropsia aviar*

ISBN Spanish edition: 978-84-92569-36-6

Translation:
BookMasters, Inc.

ISBN: 978-84-92569-84-7
D.L.: Z 1451-2012

Design, layout and printing:
Servet editorial - Grupo Asís Biomedia, S.L.
www.grupoasis.com
info@grupoasis.com

GRUPO asis

**Servet is the publishing house of Grupo Asís**



Warning:

Veterinary science is constantly evolving, as are pharmacology and the other sciences. Inevitably, it is therefore the responsibility of the veterinary surgeon to determine and verify the dosage, the method of administration, the duration of treatment and any possible contraindications to the treatments given to each individual patient, based on his or her professional experience. Neither the publisher nor the author can be held liable for any damage or harm caused to people, animals or properties resulting from the correct or incorrect application of the information contained in this book.

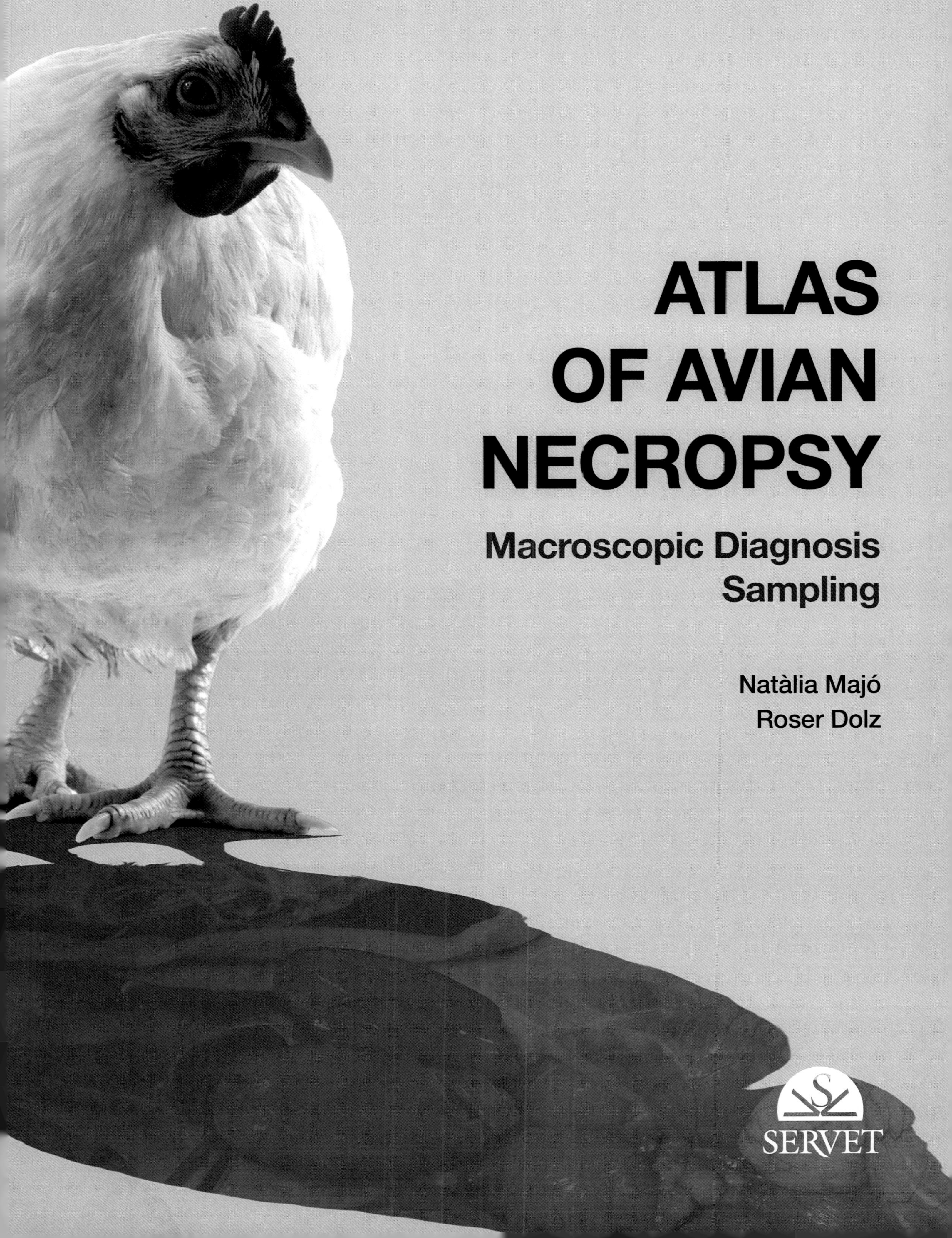

# ATLAS OF AVIAN NECROPSY

## Macroscopic Diagnosis
## Sampling

Natàlia Majó
Roser Dolz

SERVET

# PREFACE

The necropsy and subsequent evaluation of gross lesions is a gold standard diagnostic tool in the veterinary profession. In the poultry sector it is also a common practice by the veterinarian on routine visits to farms. However, little information exists on how to perform a necropsy on a bird to maximize the diagnostic yield of this procedure.

The main aim of this book is to serve as a guide both to poultry sector veterinarians and veterinary students, regarding necropsy techniques, evaluation of gross lesions and sampling. We hope the presentation of a large number of images will greatly facilitate understanding and usability of the text.

The first part of the book details the avian necropsy technique; individual organ examination; organs and systems; and their appearance when there is no type of lesion. Next, various gross lesions as well as some microscopic lesions relevant to avian pathology are presented and these are grouped by organs or by systems. Finally, guidelines are given as to sampling during a necropsy, to enable posterior diagnostic tests.

We sincerely hope that this book will be useful to all professionals related to the avian world.

**The authors**

Bellaterra (Barcelona), December 2010

# ACKNOWLEDGMENTS

Many of the images included in this book are taken from the collection of images held by the Unidad de Histología y Anatomía Patológica de la Facultad de Veterinaria de la Universitat Autònoma de Barcelona. Therefore, our sincere thanks to the teachers, interns and residents who, for many years, have collaborated by generating the photographs to improve this collection.

We also would like to express our deepest appreciation for the trust placed in us over the years by all the technicians, clinicians and veterinarians in the poultry sector, who have referred clinical cases which have allowed us to see and learn many things together. Without their cooperation it would not have been possible to produce this book, so they all may be considered co-authors of this work.

Finally, we would like to give our most special thanks to all the veterinarians and clinicians who have worked directly with us, allowing us the right of use of some of the images found here. Without their help this work would have been incomplete:

- Dr. H.L. Shivaprasad, University of California (figs. 7 and 15).
- Dr. Mercè Roca, Laboratorios Hipra (figs. 135 and 136).
- Dr. Albert Pagès, Laboratorios Hipra (fig. 119).
- Mr. Rafael Campos, poultry veterinary consultant (figs. 58, 60, 61, 64 and 66).
- Ms. Pilar Creus, Serveis Veterinaris Oficials d'Escorxador (SVOE) del Vallès Occidental (fig. 13).
- Mr. Jesús Vicente, Nanta, S.A. (figs. 25 and 80).
- Mr. Climent Faus, Elanco (figs. 5 and 6).
- Mr. Óscar Pérez, Piensos el Horreo (figs. 125 and 126).

**The authors**

Bellaterra (Barcelona), December 2010

# AUTHORS

## Natàlia Majó and Roser Dolz

Dr. Natàlia Majó is a Professor at the Teaching Unit of Histology and Pathology, Faculty of Veterinary Medicine, Universitat Autònoma de Barcelona with a Graduate degree from the European College of Veterinary Pathology (ECVP), and develops her research at the Research Centre in Animal Health (CReSA).

Dr. Roser Dolz is currently a researcher at the CReSA.

They both have Master's degrees and doctorates in Veterinary medicine from the Universitat Autònoma de Barcelona, and for more than 15 years they have been responsible for avian pathology diagnosis in the Diagnostic Service of Veterinary Pathology, Faculty of Veterinary Medicine. Furthermore, their research focuses on the study of avian viral infections, especially avian infectious bronchitis, Gumboro disease, swollen head syndrome and avian influenza. They have spoken at various national and international poultry and virology conferences, and they use their extensive clinical experience to teach avian necropsy and pathology courses, thereby participating in the ongoing education of poultry and veterinary technicians.

**Centre de Recerca en Sanitat Animal (CReSA)**
Edifici CReSA - Campus de la UAB
08193 Bellaterra (Barcelona)
www.cresa.cat

**Departament de Sanitat i d'Anatomia Animals**
Facultat de Veterinària
Universitat Autònoma de Barcelona
08193 Bellaterra (Barcelona)

# TABLE OF CONTENTS

## 1 NECROPSY TECHNIQUE IN POULTRY

# 2 MACROSCOPIC EVALUATION OF THE ORGANS

# 3 SAMPLING AND OTHER GENERAL CONSIDERATIONS

CHAPTER 1

# NECROPSY TECHNIQUE IN POULTRY

# Previous aspects to keep in mind

## Objectives of the necropsy

Necropsy is probably performed more often on poultry than on any other species, as the large number of these animals on a farm allows various birds to be allocated for this purpose, and due to their size, it is relatively easy to perform a necropsy in any farm area For this reason, poultry clinicians and technicians perform necropsies very frequently, almost daily.

The objective of performing a necropsy may be varied. The usual reason is **to determine the cause of disease and/or death in animals**. Therefore, by evaluating the medical history provided through the farmer's records and the farm registers, together with the information obtained from the necropsy, an orientative or definitive diagnosis can be developed.

When the lesions observed in the necropsy are characteristic of a particular pathology, they are known as pathognomonic lesions. In such cases, the clinical history and gross lesions observed at the necropsy are enough to establish a diagnosis. When the lesions seen during the necropsy can be found in more than one pathology, a clinical suspicion could lead towards a group of pathologies which may be included in a list of differential diagnoses. In this case, complementary laboratory techniques are needed to confirm or rule out different suspicions. Therefore, a second objective of the necropsy is to **obtain samples**, either to confirm a particular clinical suspicion or within a system of monitoring a specific pathology or treatment.

Obviously, performing the necropsy together with sampling to detect etiologic agents also **allows a better understanding of the disease**, by defining the lesions it produces and its relation to certain causative agents. Finally, the necropsy may be useful within the **legal system** when in this case the clinician acts as an expert. The information obtained at the necropsy is an important point in the final ruling drawn up by the judiciary.

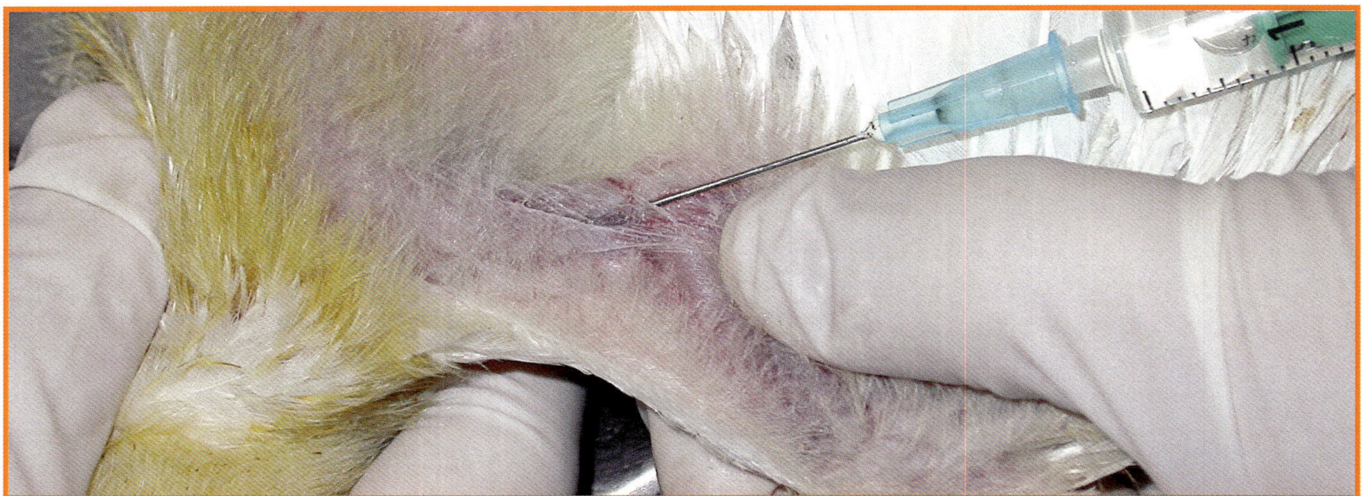

Fig. 1 | Euthanasia injection into the blood vessels of the wing.

## Selection of animals for necropsy

The concept of population diseases is used when working with production species. The objective, therefore, is not to determine the cause of death of an 'individual' animal but rather of the population of birds on a farm or poultry site. This emphasizes the extreme importance to be placed on the correct selection of the birds for necropsy, as they will affect the accurate evaluation of the gross lesions as well as the quality of the samples to be obtained, if necessary. First, they must be representative of the clinical picture observed on the farm. The necropsies should not be performed on birds which occasionally show an individual clinical process, or on cull birds considered as part of the usual farm process due to differing causes (e.g. lameness, trauma, malformations, growth retardation for various reasons, etc.).

Secondly, neither sick nor dead birds are a first choice for necropsy, since the autolysis process is very rapid in birds causing tissue changes, which may not only lead to misinterpreting nonexistent lesions, but also to prevent a correct subsequent evaluation by histology or microbiology. By way of example, a bird's gastrointestinal tract is not analysable 4 hours post mortem. The ideal situation is to choose live birds in which the clinical signs observed are representative of the clinical picture that affects the flock and perform the necropsy as soon as possible after slaughter.

## Methods of euthanasia

Today there is strict legislation regarding methods of euthanasia of animals kept for food production and used for experimental and other scientific purposes. According to the European Directive 86/609/EEC, the primary criteria to be referring to animal welfare at slaughter, are the following:

1. It must be painless.
2. The animal must achieve rapid unconsciousness and death.
3. The method must require minimum animal restraint.
4. It should avoid excitement of the animal.
5. It should be appropriate for the age, species and health of the animal, minimising possible fear and psychological stress.
6. It should be reliable, reproducible, irreversible and simple to administer (in small doses if possible).
7. It should be safe for the personnel.
8. As far as possible, it should be aesthetically acceptable for the personnel.

The method of choice in poultry is an anaesthetic overdose (sodium pentobarbital, 80 mg/kg) into the wing vein (fig. 1). If the adequate product is not available, the method of choice is cervical dislocation. This is probably the most usual slaughter method for an on-farm necropsy. The animal should be held with one hand, and with the other hand the cervical region is compressed until the atlantooccipital joint is disarticulated.

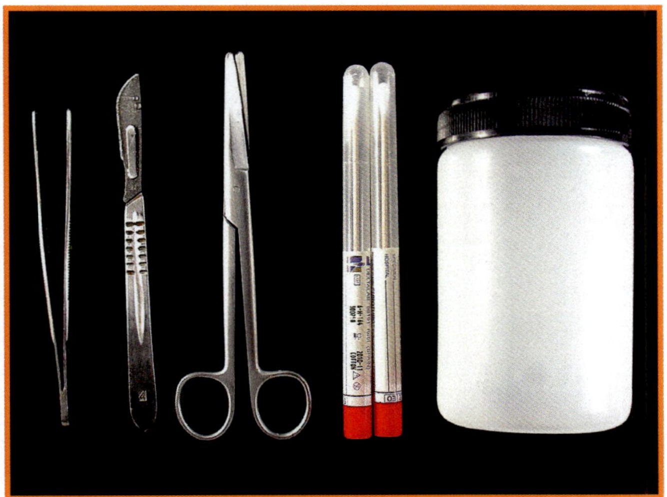

Fig. 2 | Image of the needed materials to perform a necropsy.

Although this is an accepted method, it is important to remember that proper training of personnel is vital, since speed and accuracy will avoid pain and suffering in the animal. Additionally, this method is only permitted in low weight birds, as the characteristics of the neck muscles in adult birds requires more force. Table 1 summarises the evaluation of different slaughter methods, as well as the methods permitted after stunning the animal and unacceptable methods.

## Necropsy equipment

Scissors and forceps (with or without teeth) are indispensable tools to perform an avian necropsy. Although not essential, a scalpel can be useful to make precise cuts in the organs and for opening the joints. Similarly, bone cutting forceps or large scissors may be helpful, especially with necropsies of adult birds. It is also advisable to prepare the basic materials for the slaughter of the animal and for collecting and preserving the different samples in advance. These material includes syringes, euthanasia products, blood or serum collection tubes, tissue bottles with formalin, sterile vials, pads, swabs and swabsticks (fig. 2).

Table 1. Agents and methods of euthanasia in birds. Recommendations based on the document published by FELASA on *Laboratory Animals* (1996) Vol. 30 (4); 293-316: Recommendations for euthanasia of experimental animals.

| AGENT | ASSESSMENT | OBSERVATIONS |
|---|---|---|
| Pentobarbital sodium | 5 | Acceptable. Intravenous administration. |
| T-61 | 4 | Requires practice: only in small birds (< 250 g). Intravenous administration. |
| $CO_2$ | 4 | Acceptable, especially in chicks. |
| Halothane, enflurane, isoflurane | 4 | Acceptable. |
| Cervical dislocation | 4 | Acceptable for small and juvenile birds (< 250 g) if the brain is then destroyed. |
| CO | 2 | Dangerous for personnel. |
| Electric stun | 1 | Dangerous for personnel. Other methods are preferable. |

| | |
|---|---|
| Acceptable in unconscious birds | Decapitation. |

| | |
|---|---|
| Unacceptable | • Fracture of neck.<br>• Exsanguination.<br>• Ether, chloroform, cyclopropane, cyanide gas, trichlorethylene, methoxyflurane, chloral hydrate.<br>• Strychnine, nicotine, magnesium sulfate, ketamine or other blocking agents. |

# Characteristics and stages of the necropsy technique

Performing a necropsy, especially in poultry, is a relatively simple procedure; yet it is advisable to follow correct protocol to achieve valid conclusions which are not misinterpreted, as discussed below.

There are probably differing procedures for performing the necropsy, but all must meet three crucial prerequisites:

- **Systematic necropsy.** This implies always performing the necropsy the same way in all cases, thereby ensuring an evaluation of the organs and structuring the findings.
- **Orderly necropsy.** This implies following a logical order within the necropsy system being carried out.
- **Complete necropsy.** It is necessary to examine all the organs and animal parts, without missing any. This is probably the most difficult aspect to apply when performing necropsies on a daily basis at farms. In many cases, a clear suspicion is formed from the clinical signs observed on the farm, and then the necropsy focuses only on a partial examination of some of the animal organs. But this action may cause changes in other organs to go unnoticed, which may become very important in the final diagnosis of the disease.

Prior to conducting the necropsy, the clinician must not only obtain a clinical history from the farmer, but must also undertake a visit to the farm and evaluate the clinical signs of the birds. This generally signifies forming a preconceived idea of what may be found. Although this is beneficial for guiding the case, it may also be harmful when evaluating the results of this necropsy. Therefore, it is advisable to perform the necropsy as though there were no clinical data of the birds, and later, make a joint interpretation of all the clinical and macroscopic data obtained.

In this sense, this book proposes the following necropsy technique, including the following steps:

1. External examination and sampling of the bird *in vivo*.
2. Preparation of the cadaver and opening the coelomic cavity.
3. Extraction of the internal organs.
4. Study and evaluation of the internal organs.
5. Study of the head: evaluation of the nasal cavity and the brain.
6. Study of the musculoskeletal system: evaluation of the nerves, joints, bones and muscles.

# External examination and sampling of the bird *in vivo*

On many occasions it is useful to collect blood from the animal before slaughter and necropsy, for serology and haematology. Just as the slaughter methods are regulated by European directives so are the blood collection methods, which pay special attention to the extraction site, the method and the total volume of blood obtained. Amounts drawn in no case should exceed 10% of the circulating volume (which in the case of birds is estimated at 60 ml/kg of live body weight).

Amongst the permitted methods, the most common is blood extraction from the blood vessels on the underside of the wing. The simplest method is by puncturing the vein with a needle or the tip of a scalpel (fig. 3) and allowing the blood to drip into a tube. When a sterile blood sample is required, it is also possible to aspirate the blood with a needle and syringe. Once extracted, the blood is emptied into a vial, with or without anticoagulant, depending on the subsequent use of the sample.

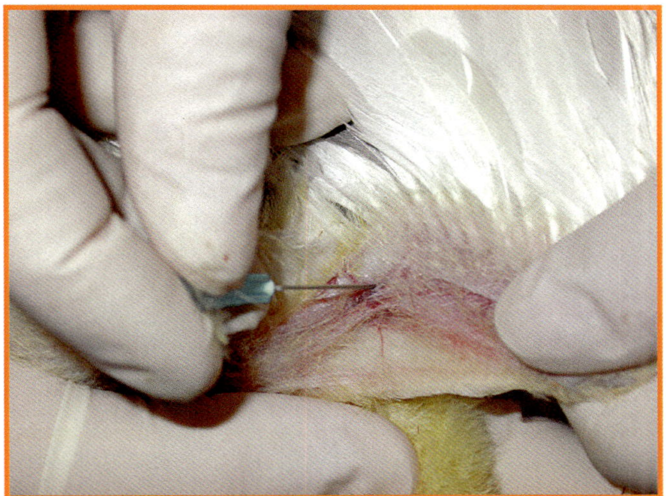

Fig. 3 | Blood collection by puncturing the vein of the wing.

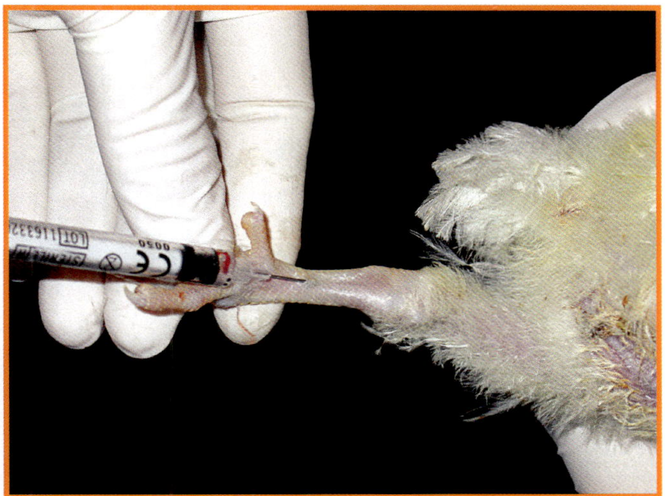

Fig. 4 | Blood collection from the leg vessels.

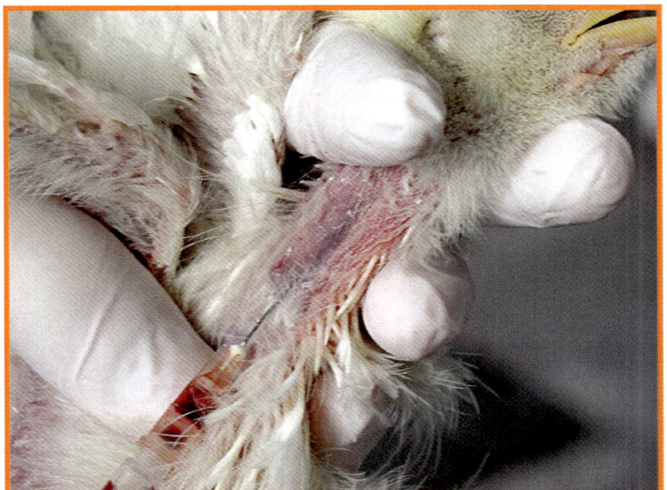

Fig. 5 | Blood collection from the jugular vein.

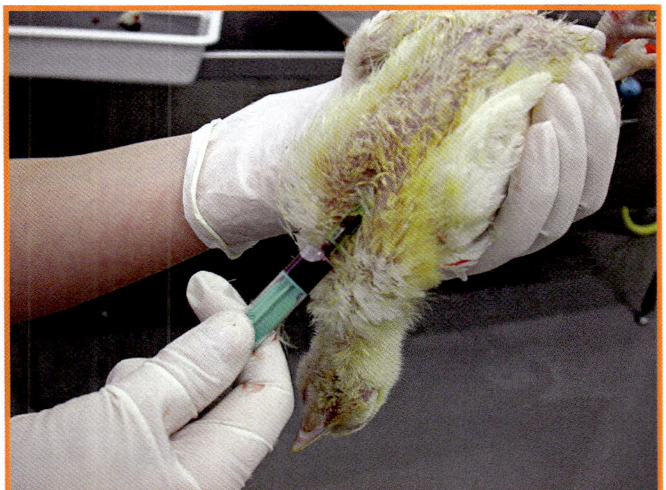

Fig. 6 | Blood collection by cardiac puncture.

Other blood extraction sites for aspirating into a syringe are the veins of the legs (fig. 4) and the jugular vein (fig. 5). This last site is particularly recommended in one-day-old chicks, where a blood sample is needed without posterior slaughter.

Finally, cardiac puncture may be the method of choice when larger volumes of blood are needed. Using this technique, the needle is inserted under the pectoral muscle until it reaches the heart (fig. 6). It is mainly used with older birds to obtain a greater volume of blood. It is important to remember that this method requires previous anaesthesia of the animal.

A complete external examination must be made before starting the necropsy (fig. 7). As discussed earlier, it is not advisable to perform a necropsy on animals that have suffered a natural death, because autolysis may produce changes.

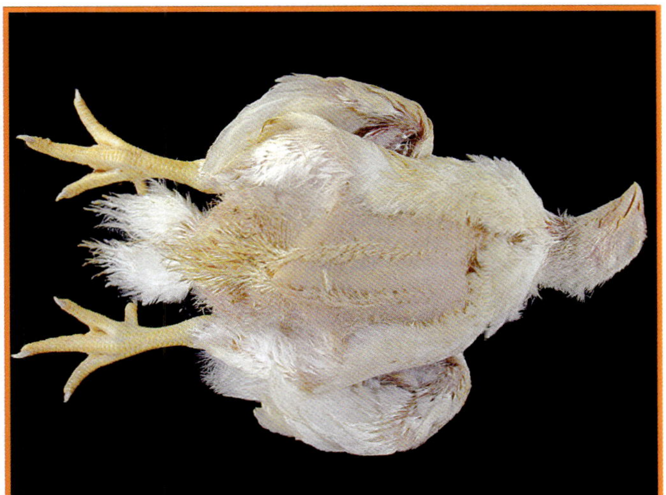

Fig. 7 | Normal external appearance of a bird. Examine the mucosa, feathers and skin of the animal.

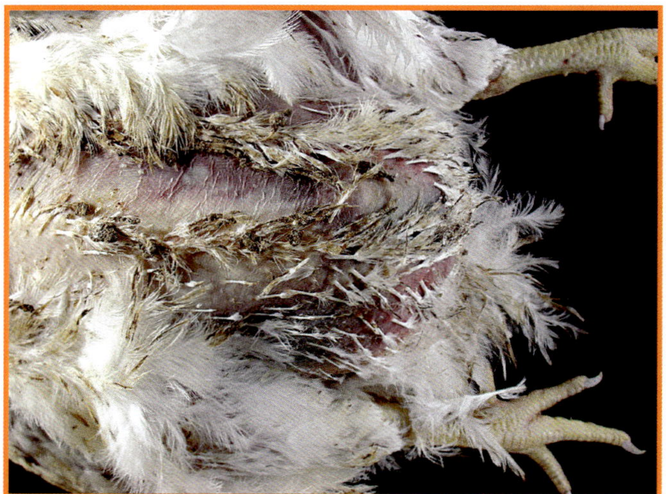

Fig. 8 | Characteristic greenish coloration of an animal in an autolytic condition.

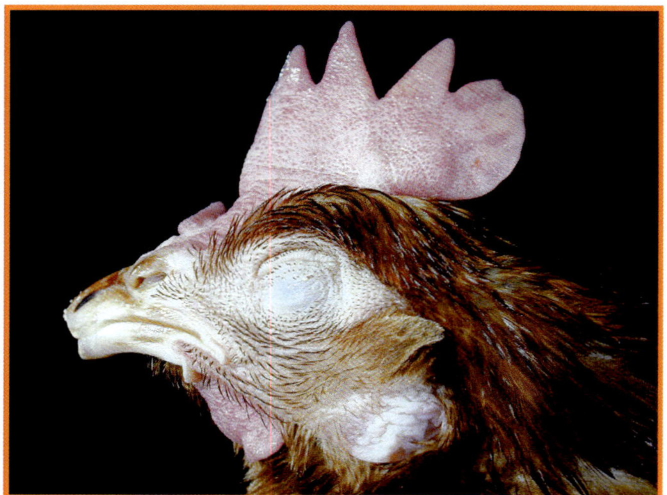

Fig. 9 | Evaluation of the coloration of the crest.

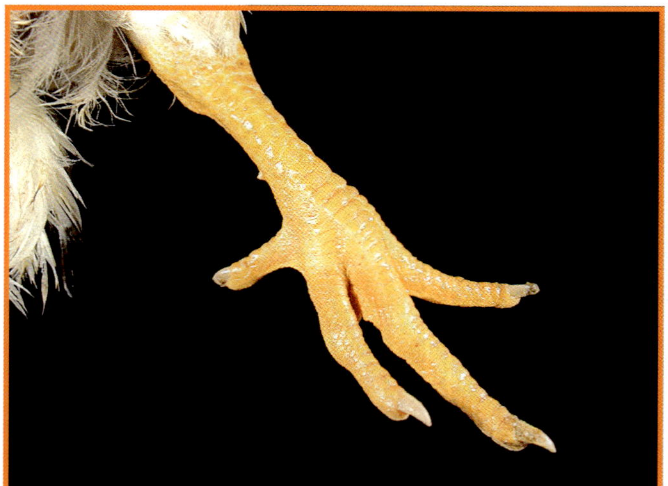

Fig. 10 | Normal coloration of the leg of a yellow pigmented broiler.

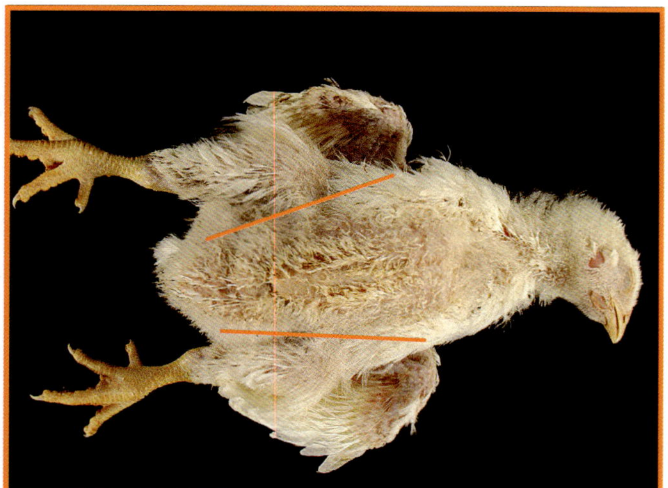

Fig. 11 | Area of incision in the animal's thigh to stabilize the cadaver.

Therefore, if there are no birds to be slaughtered, this external examination must also determine the extent and degree of changes in the cadaver. This will establish the time that has elapsed since the death of the animal and the state of decomposition of the cadaver. Birds with an advanced state of autolysis (fig. 8) should be discarded from subsequent necropsy.

The external examination should be initiated at the head region. Assess the appearance of the comb and wattles, paying special attention to its coloration and the presence of scabs or traumatic lesions (fig. 9). Also examine the eye region, namely the opacity of the ocular conjunctiva and presence of possible exudates, as well as possible changes in the periorbital and infraorbital sinuses. Then examine the ear and nasal openings, pressing lightly to detect the presence of exudates. Open the beak to assess the oral cavity and the tongue. It is very important to examine the state of the plumage and ensure that the feathers are clean and uniformly distributed. Lastly, assess the cloacal region, both the mucosa as well as the appearance of feathers around the cloacal opening, and the coloration of the legs, both their colour and by touching the skin that covers the tibiofemoral region (fig. 10).

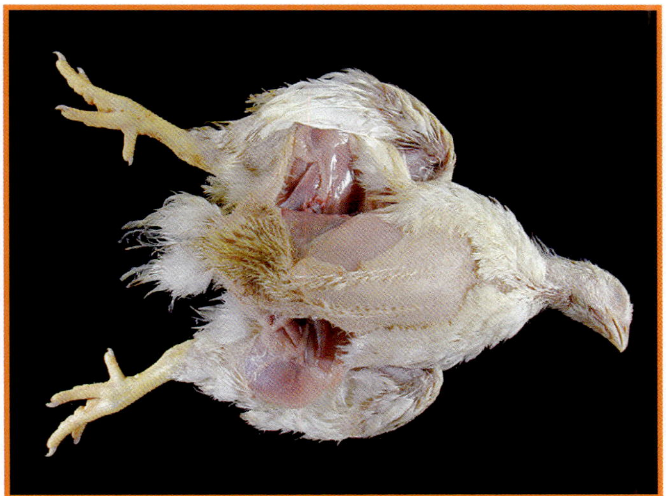

Fig. 12 | Posterior extremities dislocated to stabilize the cadaver.

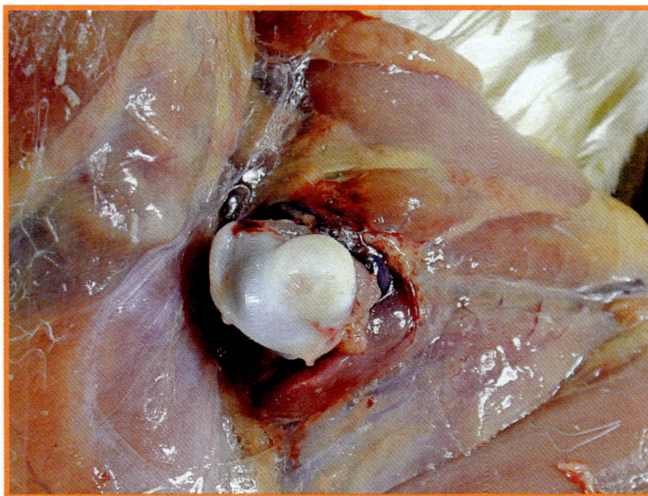

Fig. 13 | Normal appearance of the femoral head once dislocated. The joint surface should be white, smooth and shiny.

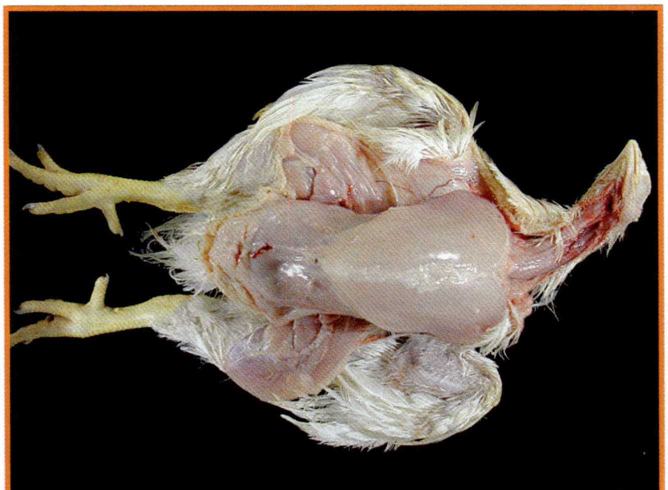

Fig. 14 | Longitudinal incision to the base of the beak to expose the pectoral muscle and neck region.

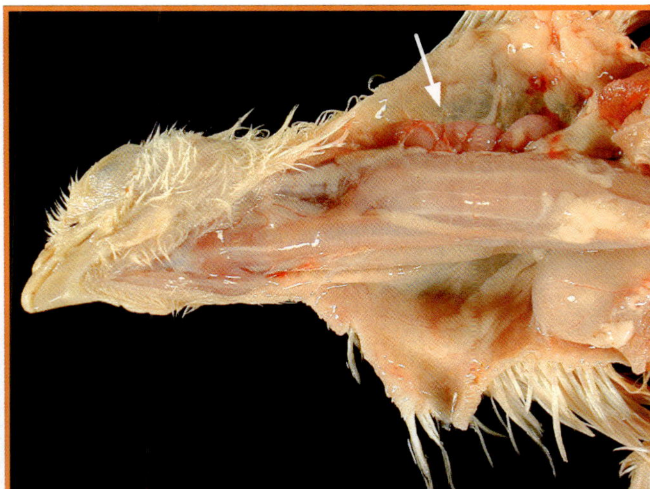

Fig. 15 | Location and normal appearance of the thymus, located laterally in the neck region (arrow).

# Preparation of the cadaver and opening the coelomic cavity

Once the external examination is finished, proceed to open the animal. The bird is placed in a dorsal decubitus position and with a scalpel or scissors two parallel cuts are made through the skin and subcutaneous tissue on each inner thigh (fig. 11) and the femoral heads are dislocated (fig. 12) to stabilise the animal. At this point, the aspect of the femoral head should be noted (fig. 13) to detect possible lesions in the femoral joints, such as femoral head necrosis.

Next, make a longitudinal incision from the base of the beak to the cloacal region, and a transverse incision below the breast. Then, reflect the skin of the animal, exposing the pectoral muscle (fig. 14). At this point evaluate the condition of the animal flesh, taking into account the volume of pectoral muscle. Evaluate the crop and its contents, as well as the thymus. The thymus is a multilobular, lymphoid organ, elongated and bilateral, that is to say, found on both sides of the neck (fig. 15). It reaches its maximum size at 17 weeks of life and involutes thereafter, so that by 20-22 weeks it is half the normal size. The examination is important to estimate the condition of the animal's immune system.

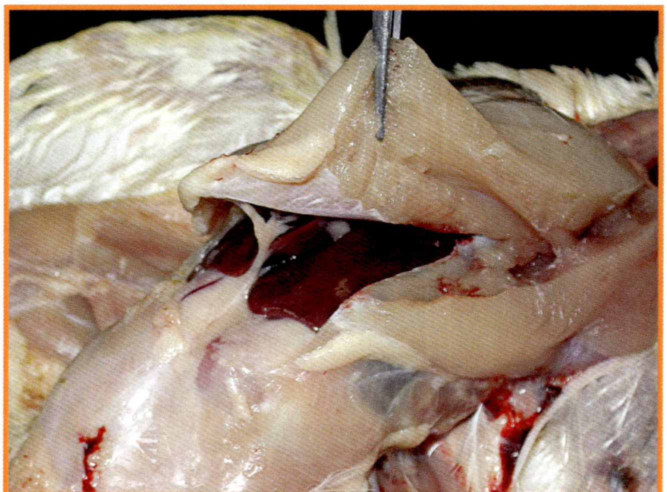

Fig. 16 | incision in the area below the breast for opening the coelomic cavity.

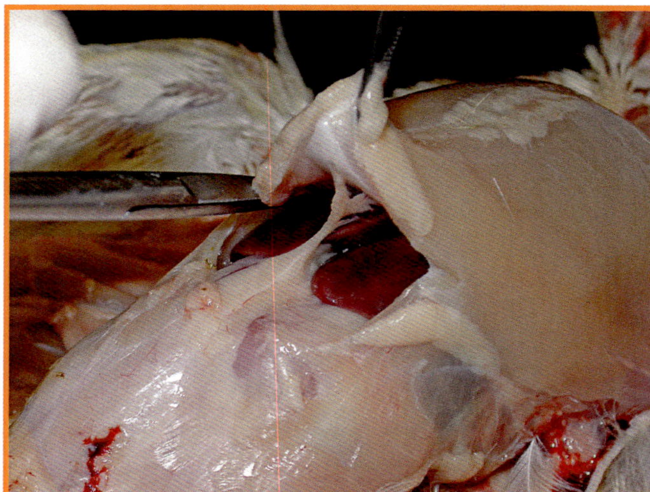

Fig. 17 | Cut of the ribs on both sides to open the coelomic cavity.

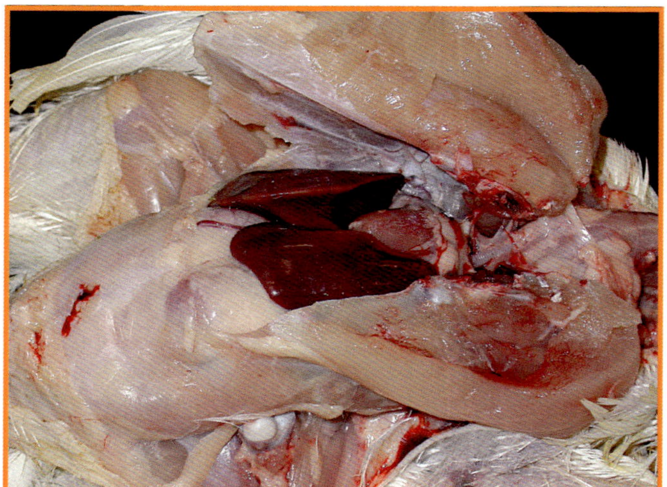

Fig. 18 | Total opening of the coelomic cavity, cutting the clavicle and coracoids.

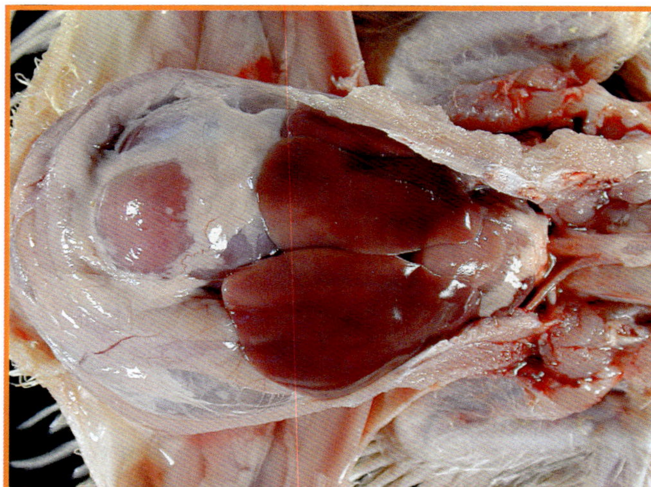

Fig. 19 | Distribution of the organs in the coelomic cavity.

Unlike mammals, birds do not have two cavities, thoracic and abdominal, but just one internal cavity called the coelomic cavity, where most of the vital organs are found. To open the coelomic cavity, make a cut in the area located below the breast using a pair of scissors (fig. 16). Next, make two small lateral cuts until reaching the ribs, and with the help of the bone cutting forceps cut the ribs (in the cranial direction) (fig. 17), the clavicle and coracoids on both sides to expose the organs of the coelomic cavity (figs. 18 and 19). This is the precise moment to assess the presence of diverse exudates and the condition of the air sacs, as on the removal of the organs these will most likely break. The air sacs in a recently slaughtered animal, must be transparent, smooth and shiny (fig. 20).

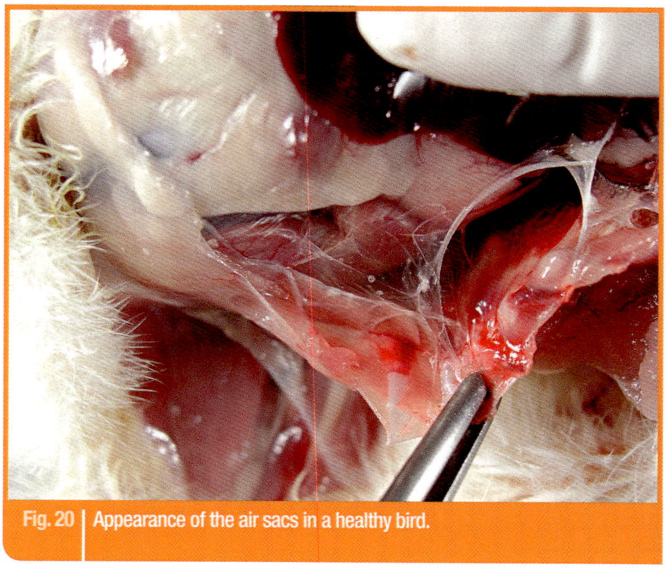

Fig. 20 | Appearance of the air sacs in a healthy bird.

# Extraction of the internal organs

The coelomic cavity organs are removed together. To achieve this, a cut is made in both commissures of the beak (fig. 21) and in both sides of the hyoid bone, exposing the oral cavity (fig. 22). An incision is made in the soft palate region (fig. 23) and the trachea and the oesophagus through to the crop are cut and removed together by gentle traction (fig. 24). Continue cutting until reaching the heart, and then again with gentle traction and helped with the tips of the scissors, separate the lungs from the dorsal region of the coelomic cavity (fig. 25). The liver and the gastrointestinal tract are extracted whole together with these organs. Simply pull gently with the hands towards the caudal region, where the rectum remains attached to the animal in the cloacal region (fig. 26). The bursa of Fabricius is located in this cloacal region, and it should be extracted with the rest of the organs from the coelomic cavity. This is a small, round lymphoid organ located in the dorsal part of the cloaca (fig. 27). Like the thymus, this organ is not present throughout the animal's life, but involutes between 14 and 20 weeks. Once the bursa is localized, a U-shaped incision is cut around it, so that most of the organs of the coelomic cavity have been removed (fig. 27).

In the case of adult hens, the reproductive system is also found in the coelomic cavity (fig. 28) which is extracted along with all the organs, as is the digestive system (fig. 29).

Only the genitourinary system will remain in the interior of the coelomic cavity, and the reproductive system (testes and oviduct) in the case of young birds (figs. 30a and 30b). Although the kidneys are examined in situ, it may be necessary to extract them for sampling. To extract the kidneys, which are totally inserted into the pelvis bones, the best system is to exert a slight pull from the medial and caudal region of the kidneys with forceps, and with the tip of the scissors to help extraction (fig. 31).

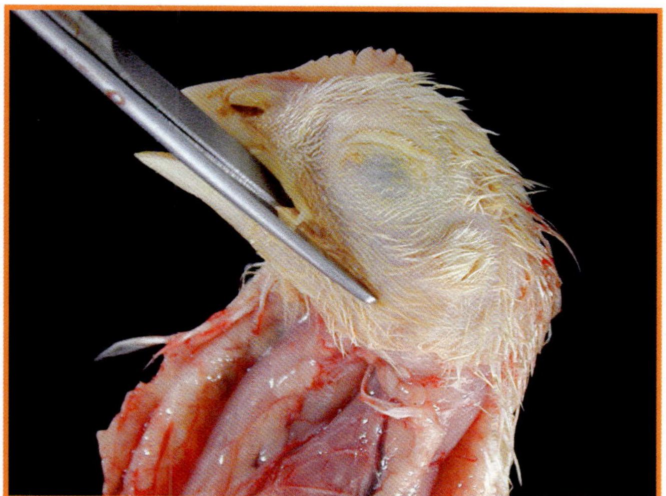

Fig. 21 | Lateral cut of the beak to remove the organs of the coelomic cavity.

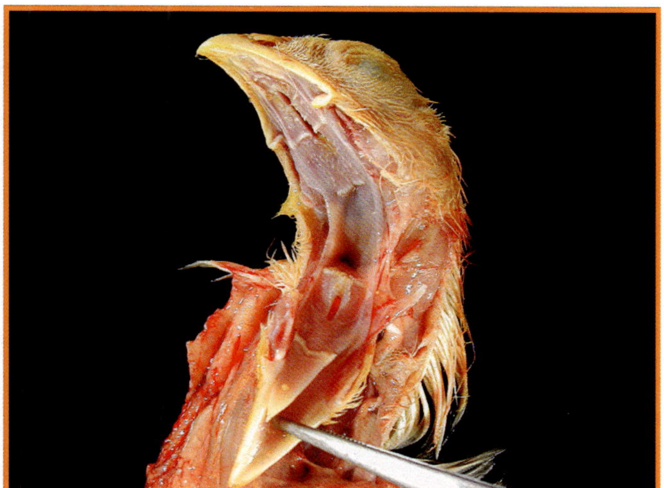

Fig. 22 | Appearance of the oral cavity after cutting the hyoid bone on both sides of the beak.

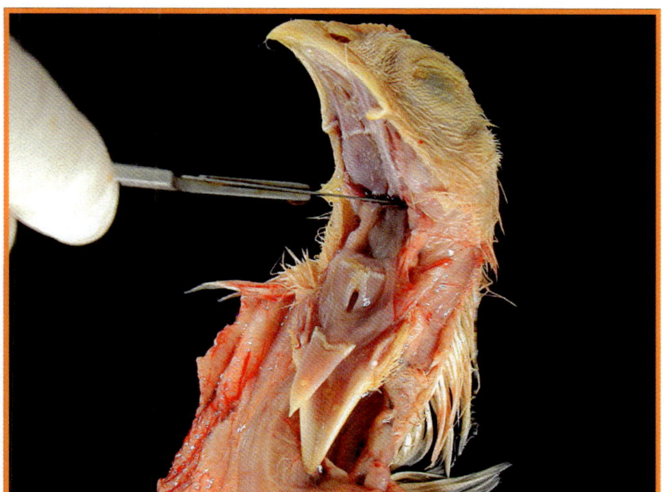

Fig. 23 | Incision in the soft palate to separate the oesophagus.

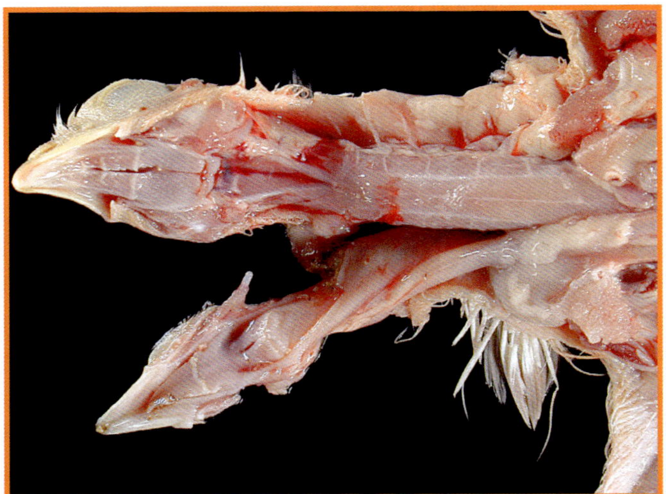

Fig. 24 | Dissection of the neck region by traction of the trachea and the oesophagus.

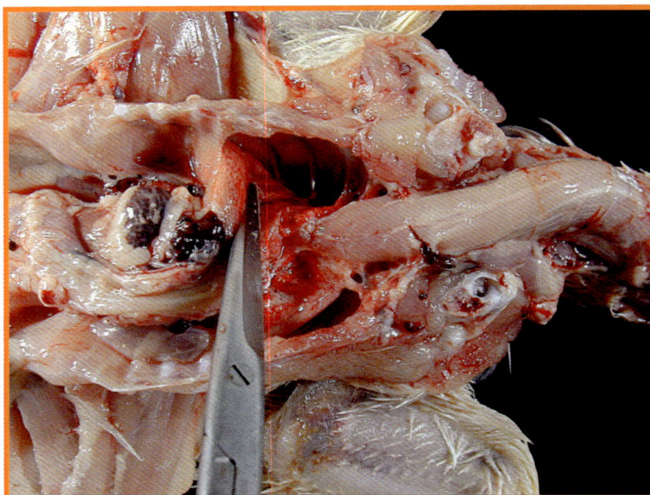

Fig. 25 | Extraction of the lungs.

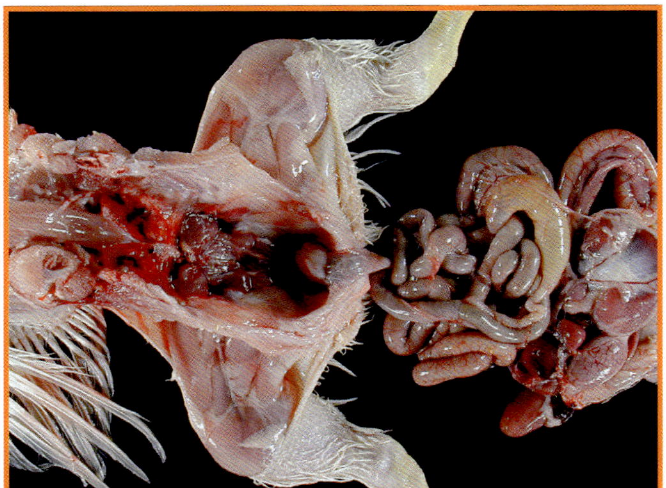

Fig. 26 | Appearance of the intestinal system and organs of the coelomic cavity, still attached to the cadaver in the cloacal region.

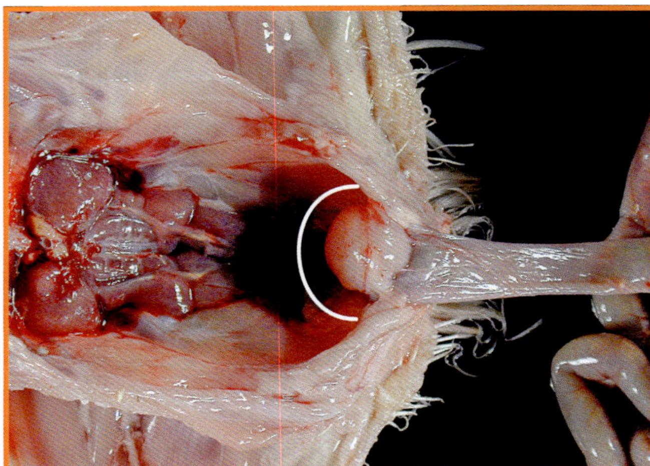

Fig. 27 | Normal appearance of the bursa of Fabricius in the cloacal region. To separate all the organs, an incision must be made around the bursa and the cloaca (line).

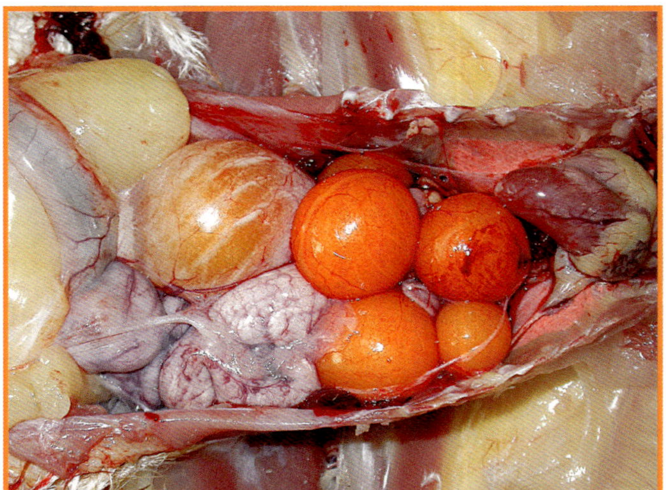

Fig. 28 | Image of the mature female reproductive system in the coelomic cavity of an adult hen, prior to extraction.

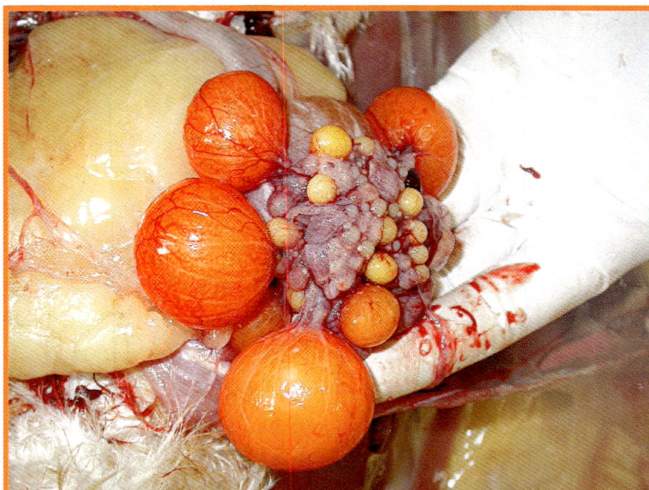

Fig. 29 | Traction of the reproductive system towards the caudal region, to extract it together with the rest of the organs of the coelomic cavity.

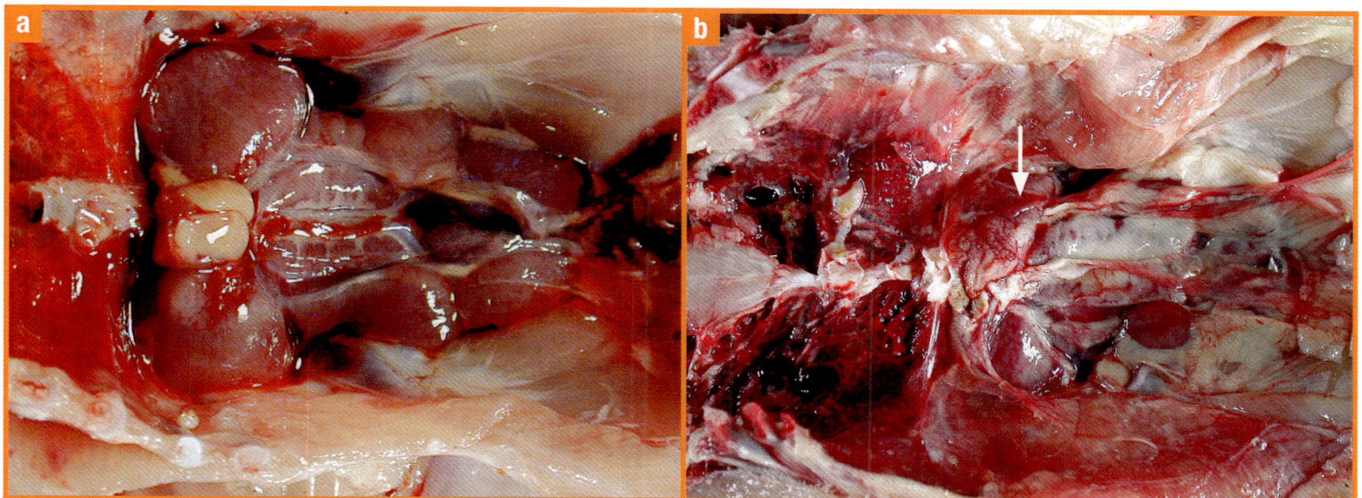

Fig. 30 | Appearance of the kidneys and testes in the coelomic cavity of a juvenile bird (a). Appearance of the kidneys and immature oviduct (arrow) in the coelomic cavity of a juvenile bird (b).

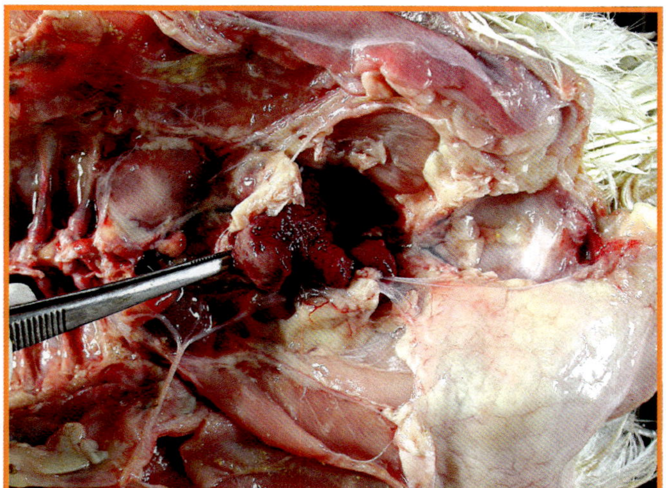

Fig. 31 | Extracting the kidneys by traction from the caudal area.

## Study and evaluation of the internal organs

The correct evaluation of the organs is performed once they are removed, by separating and opening them completely. First, make a cut at the entrance of the proventriculus to separate the ventral side of the beak, the trachea, the oesophagus, the crop, the heart and the lungs from the rest of the visceral organs (figs. 32a and 32b).

To examine this group of visceral organs it is not necessary to separate them individually.

The oesophagus and the crop are separated from the trachea, leaving them connected at the most caudal area (fig. 33) and then opened longitudinally to evaluate the appearance of the mucosal surfaces (fig. 34). Also open the trachea longi-

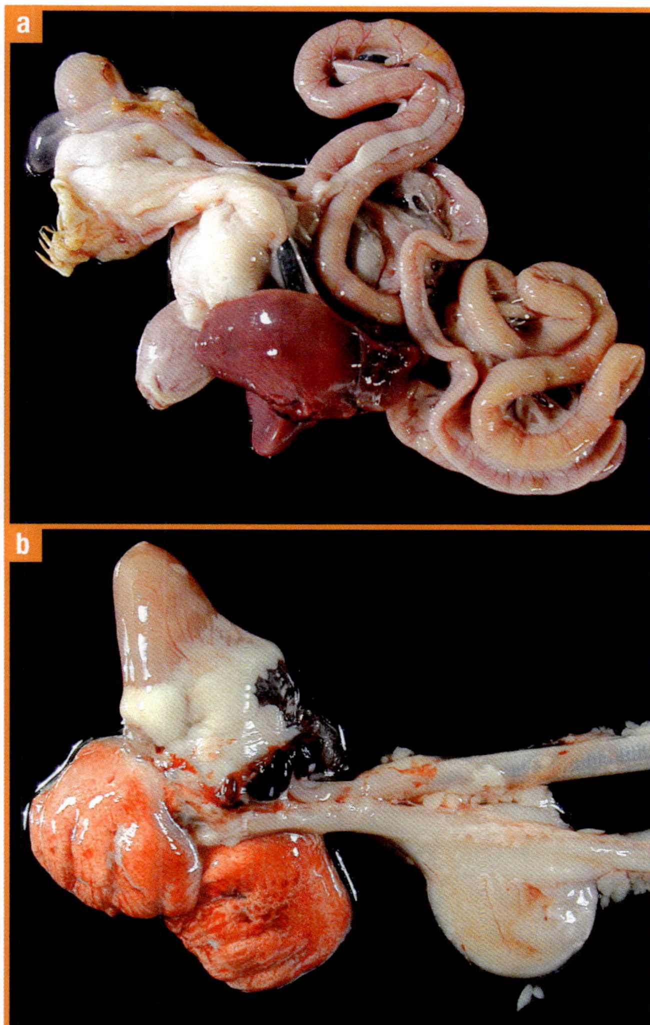

Fig. 32 | Intestinal tract grouped together with the liver, spleen and bursa of Fabricius after its extraction from the coelomic cavity (a). Appearance of the lungs, heart, crop, trachea and oesophagus once separated from the rest of the organs (b).

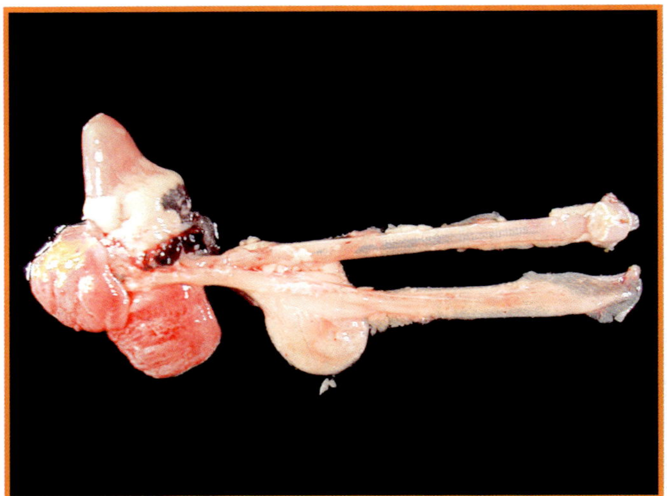
Fig. 33 | Separation of the oesophagus from the cranial region of the trachea, for its subsequent opening.

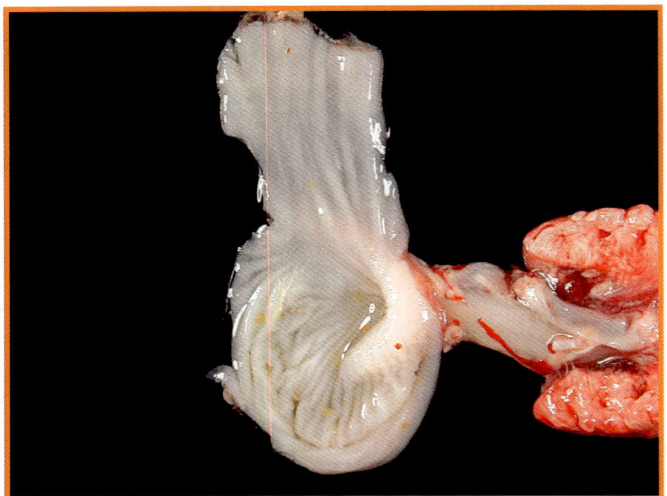
Fig. 34 | A longitudinal cut to open the oesophagus and the crop.

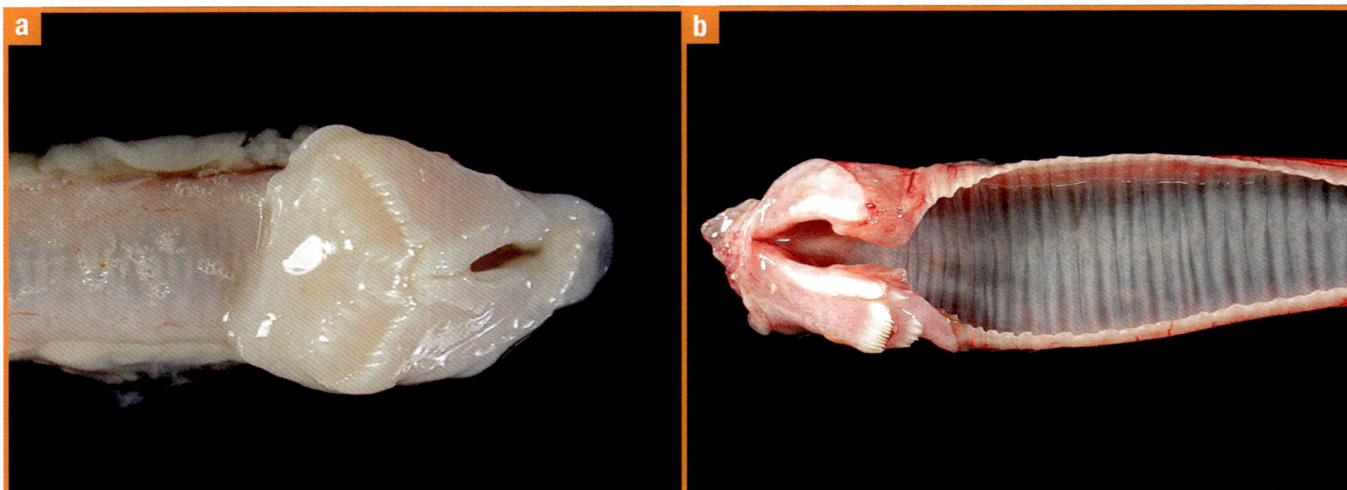
Fig. 35 | Appearance of the larynx in the cranial area of the trachea (a). Longitudinal section of the trachea (b).

tudinally to the bronchi, to examine the appearance of the mucosa and the presence of exudates in the tracheal lumen. (figs. 35a and 35b). The coloration of the lungs should be pinkish, although it must be noted that the diagnostic value of this observation may be low, especially in animals found dead or badly bled (fig. 36). The texture must also be evaluated along with the presence of areas of consolidation. Lastly, open the pericardial sac and examine the heart. Make a transverse section to evaluate the myocardial wall and the ventricular cavities, which in birds are practically virtual (figs. 37a and 37b).

Then separate the spleen, the liver, the proventriculus and gizzard, and the intestinal loops. Examine the size, appearance and colour of the serosa of the spleen and liver, and

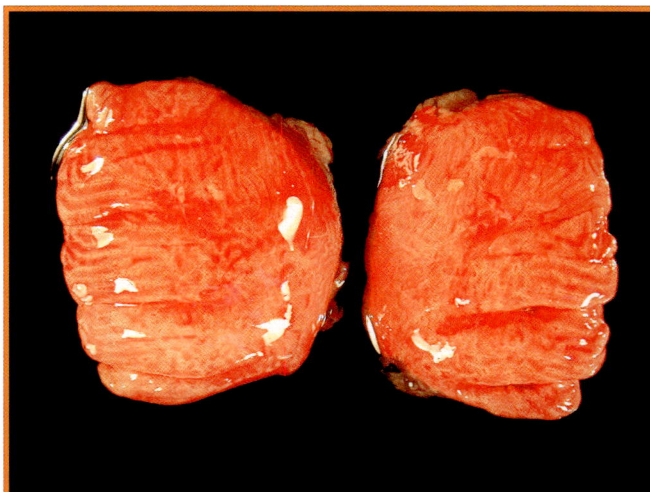
Fig. 36 | Appearance of the lungs of a healthy bird.

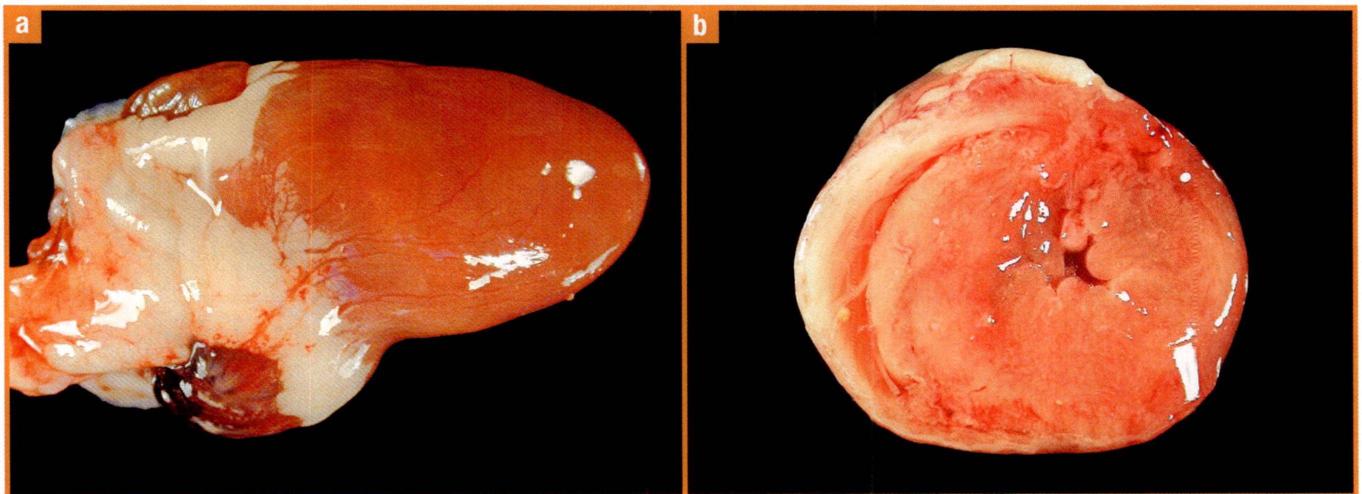

Fig. 37 | Appearance of the heart after cutting the pericardial sac (a). Transversal cut of the heart to assess the wall thickness and the size of the ventricular cavities (b).

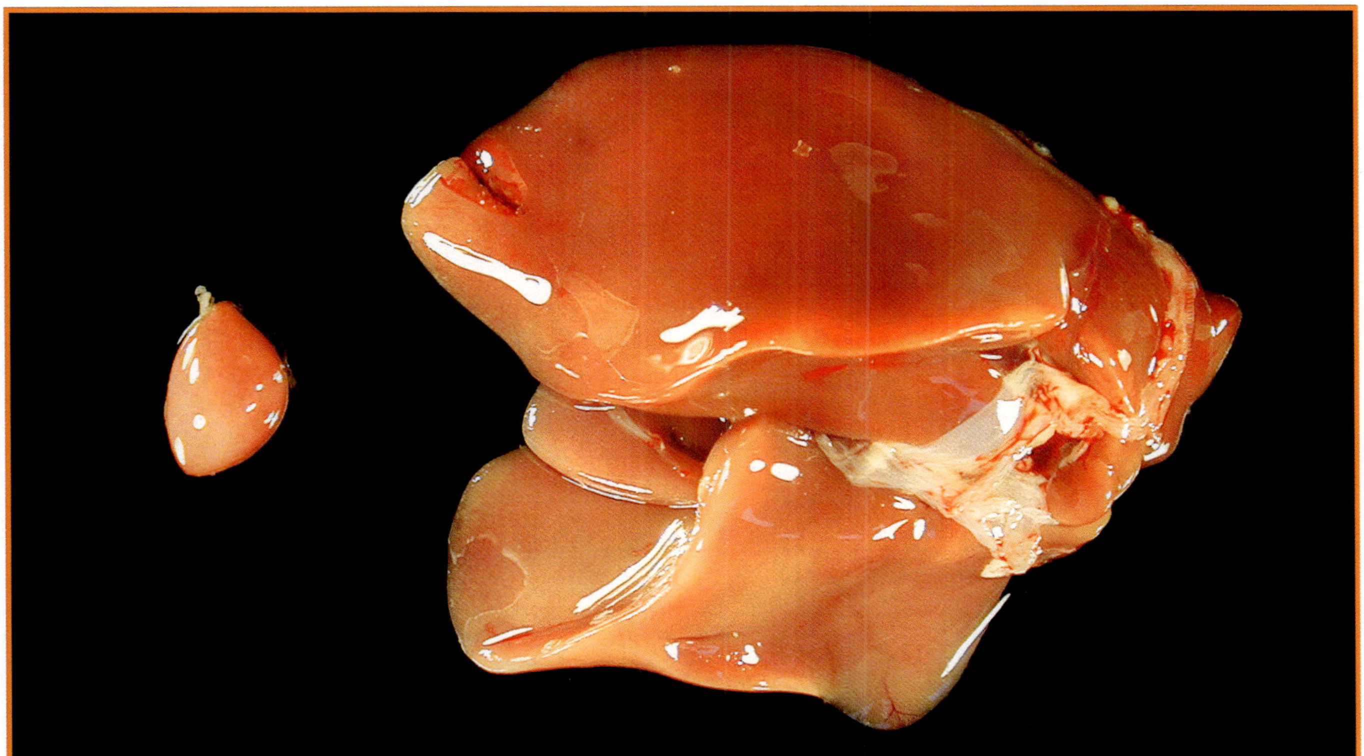

Fig. 38 | Normal appearance of the liver and spleen.

finally cut into the parenchyma to examine its texture and hardness (fig. 38). Open the proventriculus and gizzard longitudinally and separate the coilin layer from the gizzard wall to observe possible erosion or ulceration (fig. 39a and 39b).

Next, separate the intestinal loops and if possible place them in an orderly manner, as to identify the different regions (fig. 40). Although this practice is difficult under field necropsy conditions, it is always necessary to identify each region to be able to localize any lesions. The most cranial region of the intestine, i.e. the one continuing from the gizzard, is the duodenal loop, and it is held and attached by the pancreas (fig. 41). Continuing from here are the jejunum and ileum that are separated anatomically by Meckel's diverticulum, point of resorption of the yolk sac during the first days of life of the chick

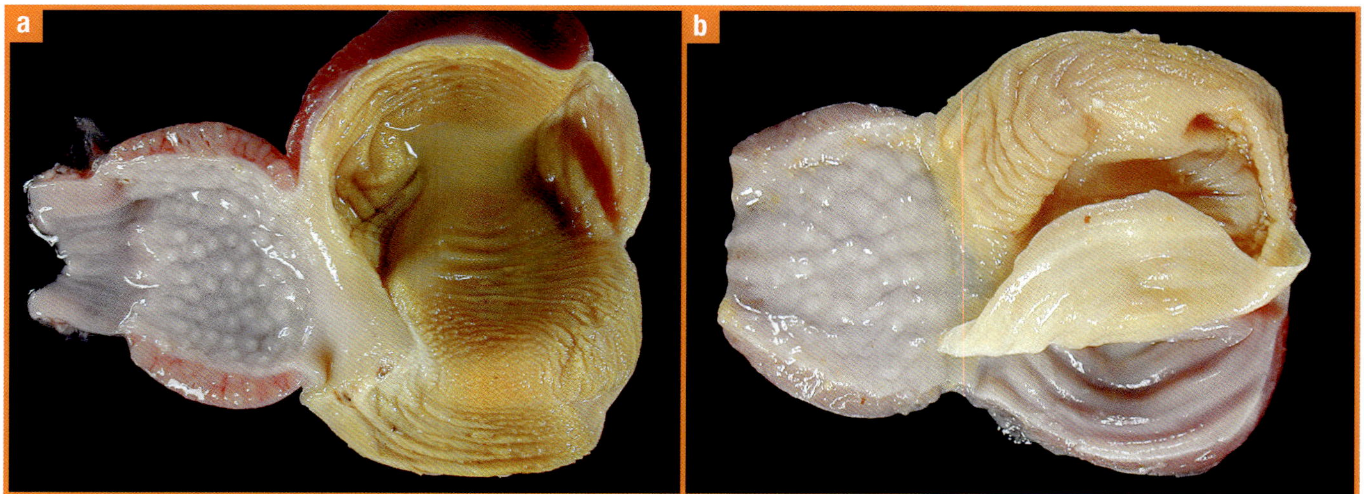

Fig. 39 | Gizzard and proventriculus after performing a longitudinal section to evaluate the mucosa of both organs (a). Separation of coilin layer covering the mucosa of the gizzard (b).

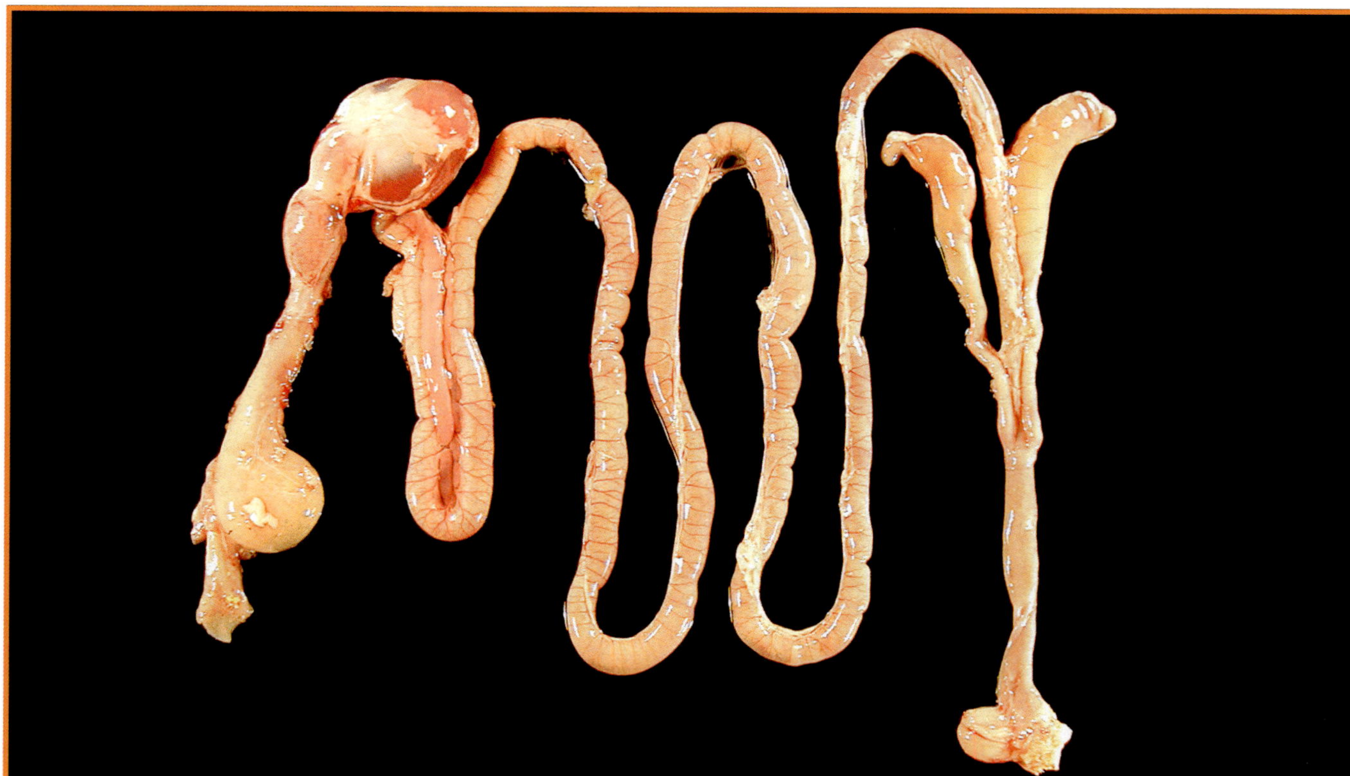

Fig. 40 | Orderly placement of the intestinal loops for their correct identification.

(fig. 42). At the end of the ileum are the ceca and finally the rectum, ending with the cloaca and the bursa of Fabricius.

To evaluate the intestine it is not enough to simply examine the serosa, but rather it is essential to open a section of each region (fig. 43). The correct evaluation of the digestive tract is based on the joint examination of intestinal contents and the appearance of the mucosa. The appearance of the intestinal content varies in different intestinal regions. In the duodenum it is fairly liquid and whitish (fig. 44) and it becomes more granular as it advances through the intestinal tract (fig. 45). In the ceca the content is paste-like and the colour ranges from orange to dark green (fig. 46). At the base of the ceca it is

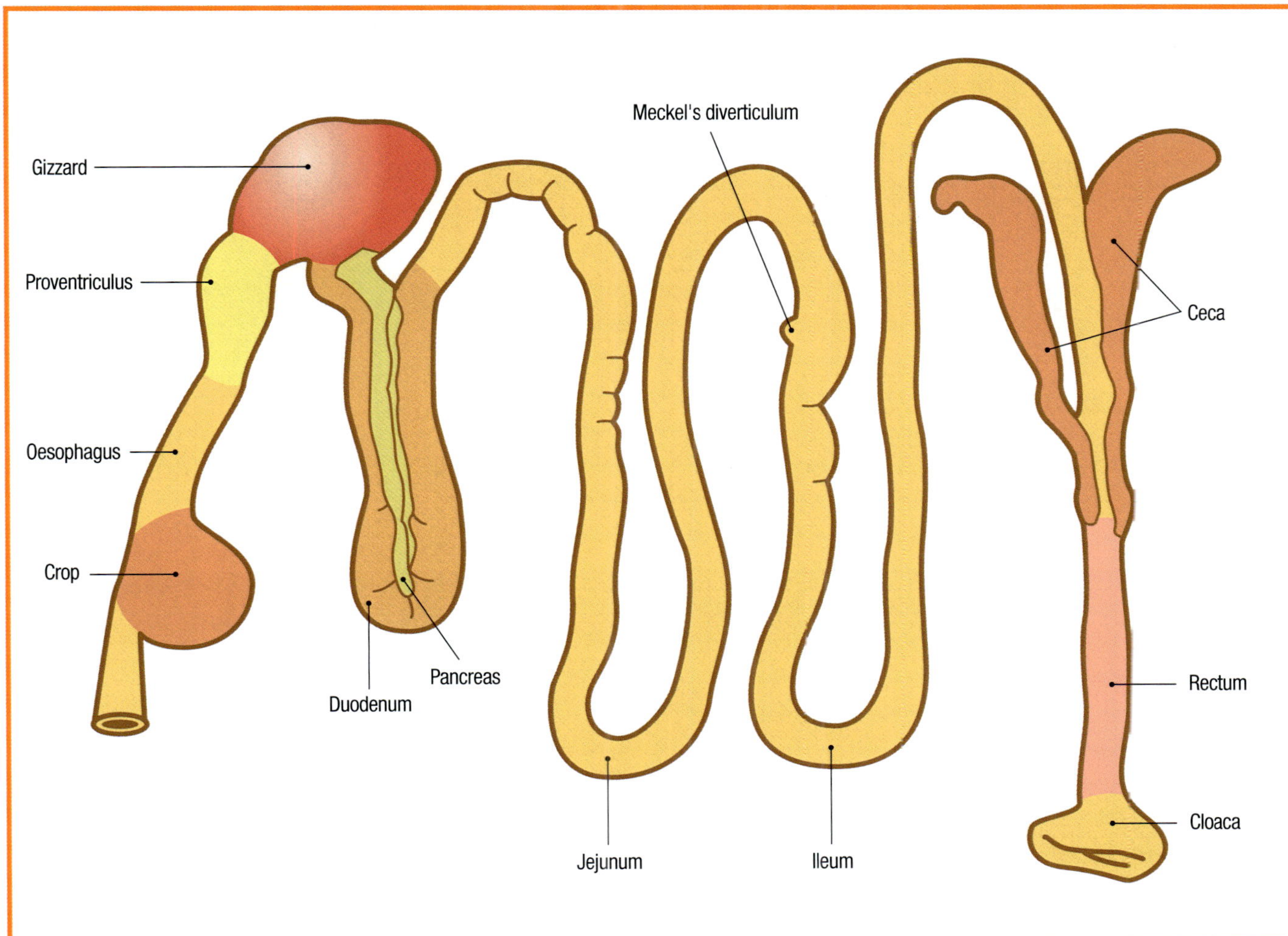


Fig. 41 | Location of each of the section of the intestine.

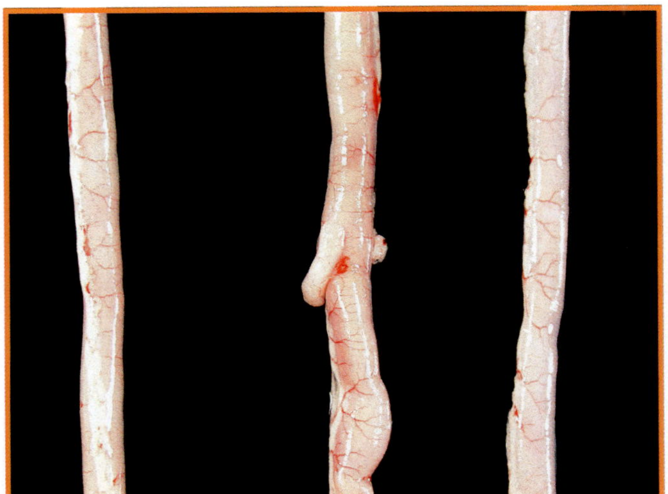

Fig. 42 | Detail of Meckel's diverticulum.

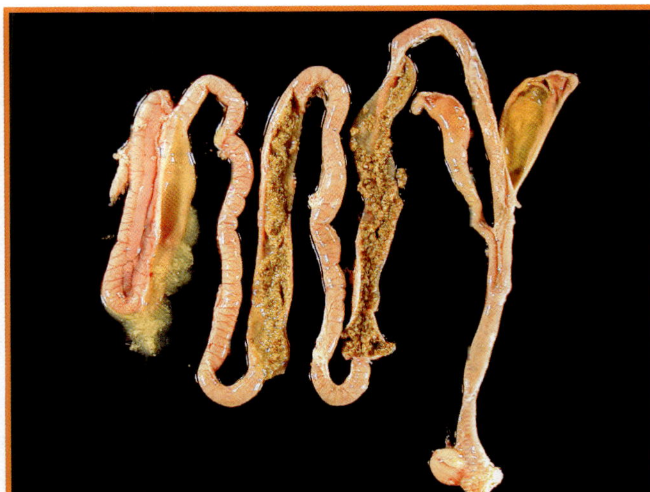

Fig. 43 | Opening various sections of the intestine in order to evaluate the appearance of the mucosa and the content.

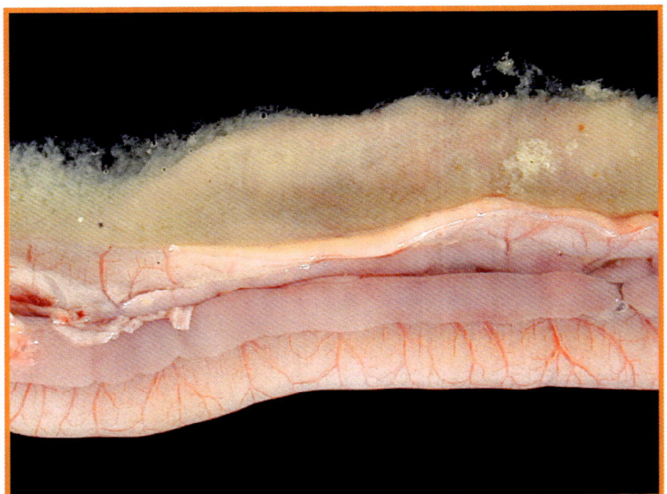

Fig. 44 | Appearance of the normal content of the duodenum.

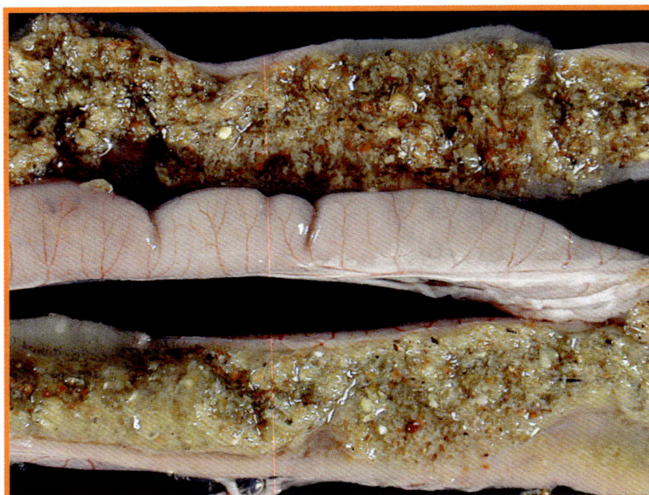

Fig. 45 | Appearance of the intestinal contents of a healthy bird.

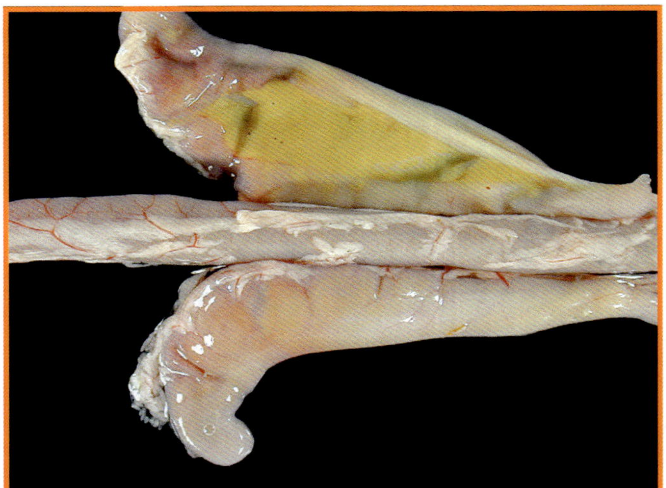

Fig. 46 | Normal appearance of the ceca.

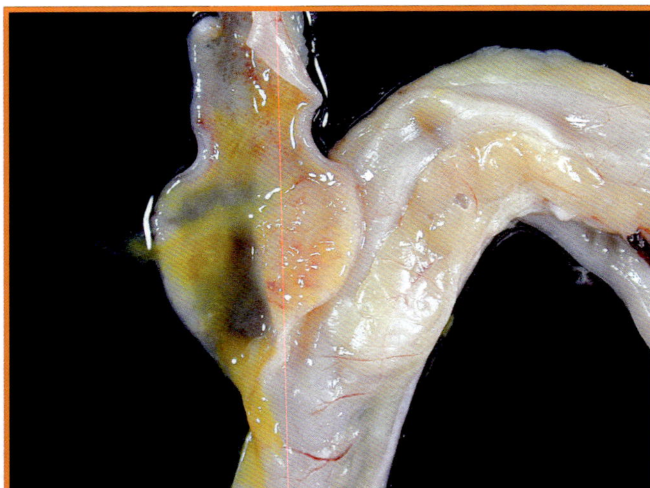

Fig. 47 | Appearance of the cecal tonsils situated in the base of the entrance to the ceca.

important to examine the cecal tonsils (fig. 47). The bursa of Fabricius is evaluated externally, by the appearance of the serosa and its size. Although this varies widely depending upon the age of the bird and the Gumboro vaccine programme, so the spleen can be used as a reference. For example, in birds of approximately 4 weeks, the spleen should be about 2/3 the size with respect to the bursa of Fabricius (fig. 48). Finally, the bursa of Fabricius is cut transversally to evaluate the mucosa (fig. 49).

The reproductive system in adult hens is extracted completely, starting with the ovary, oviduct and it is incised where it connects to the cloaca (figs. 50a and 50b). Once removed from the animal, it is opened longitudinally and the condition of the mucosa is examined in the different parts of the oviduct

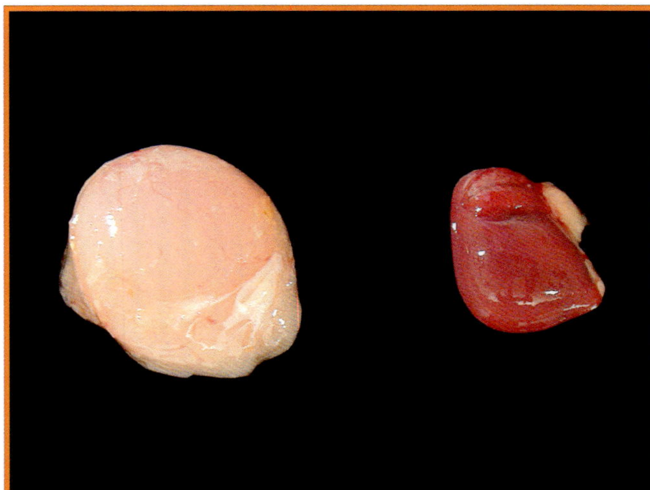

Fig. 48 | Comparative size of the spleen and the bursa of Fabricius belonging to the same animal.

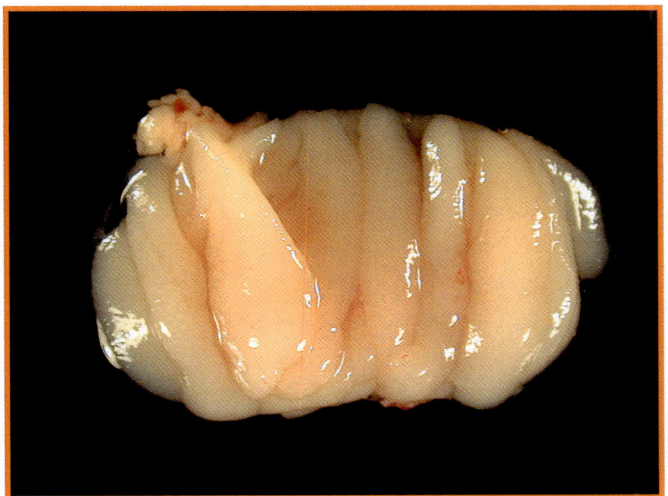

Fig. 49 | Appearance of the folds and mucosa of the bursa of Fabricius, after opening with a longitudinal incision.

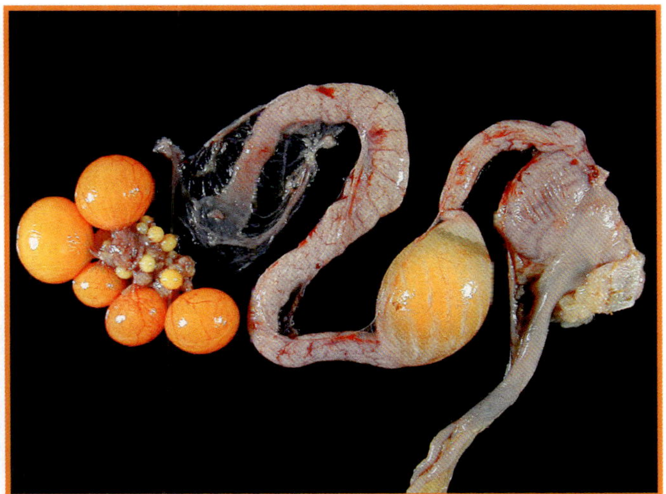

Fig. 50a | Normal appearance of the reproductive system of the hen, after removing it from the coelomic cavity.

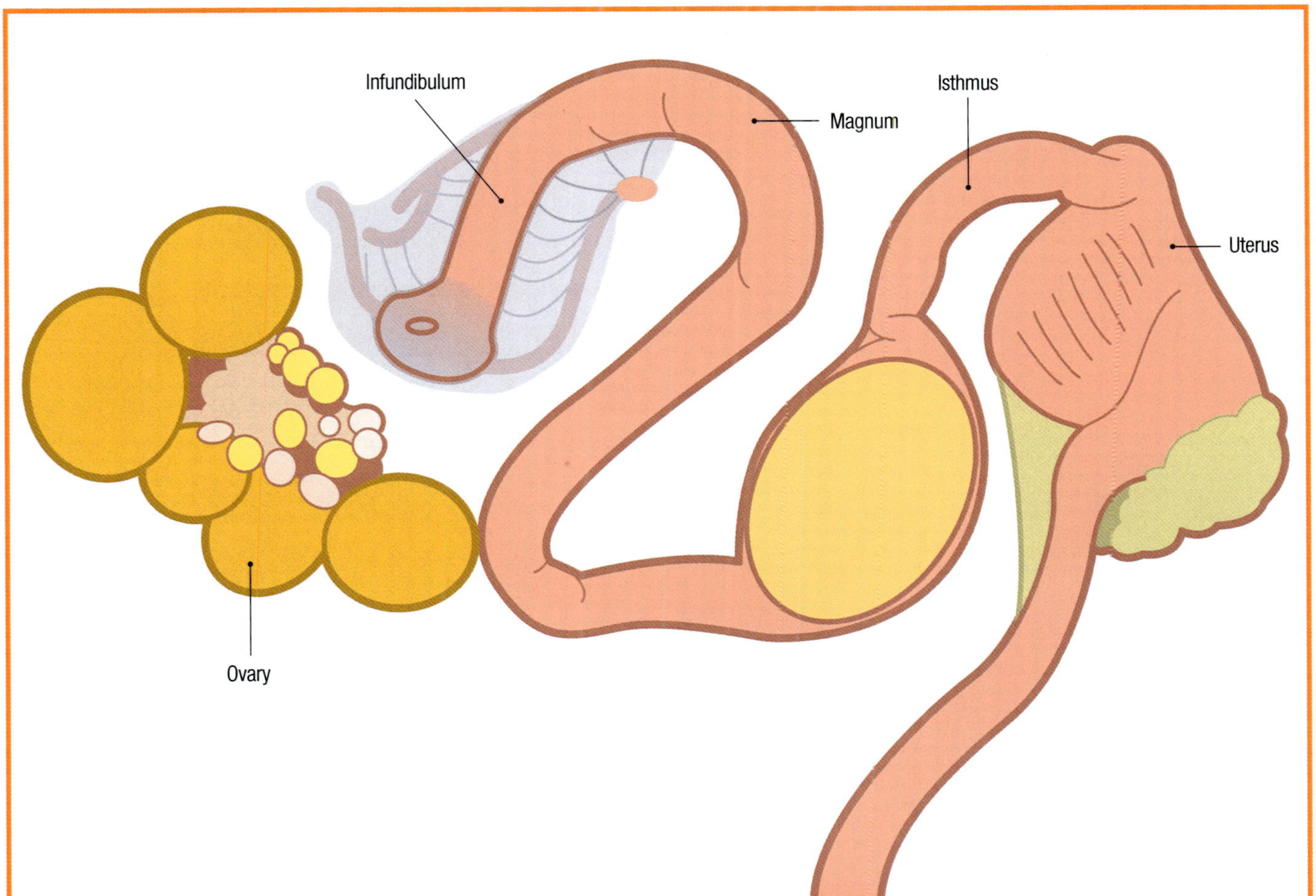


Fig. 50b | Reproductive system regions of the hen.

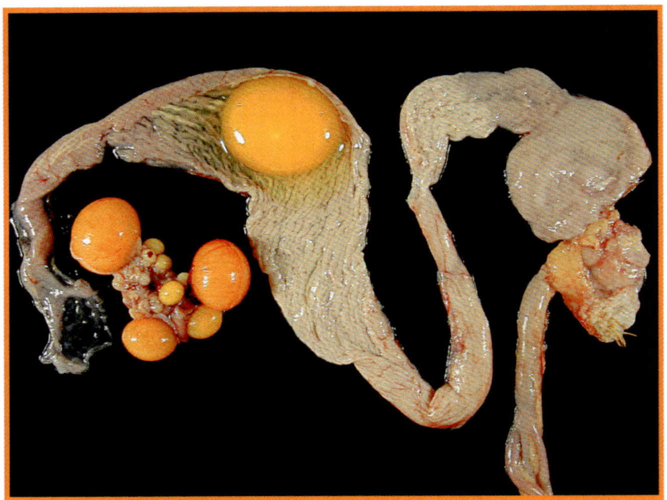

Fig. 51 | Appearance of the mucosa from the different sections of the hen's reproductive system once opened.

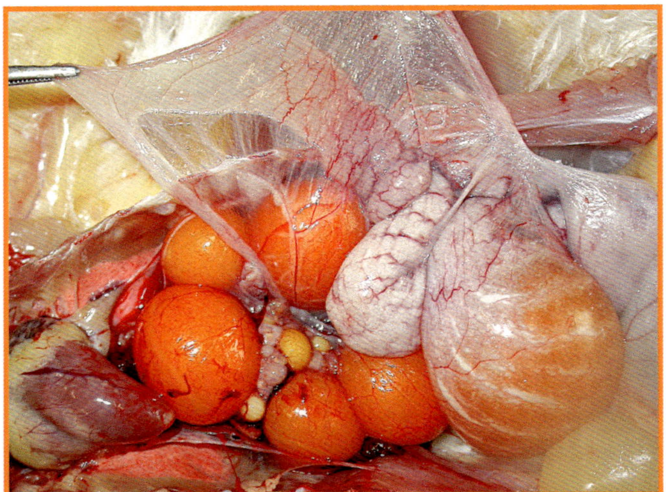

Fig. 52 | Appearance of the striated portion and tubular portion of the infundibulum.

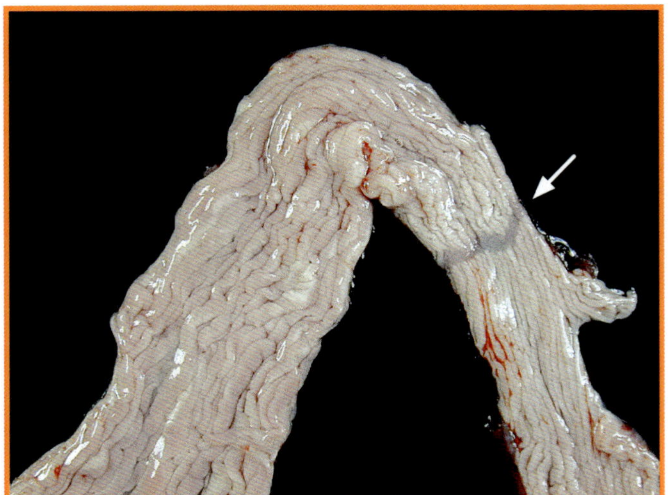

Fig. 53 | Image of the glandular band which separates the magnum from the isthmus regions (arrow).

(fig. 51). In hens only the left-side ovary and oviduct develop, the right-side remains atrophied. In the ovary, examine the number of ova and their stage of development. There should be at least five large-sized follicles at different stages of development which will be the next five ova to ovulate. Then, at the most cranial region of the oviduct is the **infundibulum**- consisting of a striated portion and a tubular portion (fig. 52). This section receives the follicles released from the ovary, the chalaza is secreted and fertilisation occurs. The ovule remains about 15 minutes in the infundibulum. The next, and probably longest, section is the **magnum**, where the egg remains for about three hours and part of the albumin is secreted. Then, the oviduct narrows into the region called the **isthmus**. Between the magnum and the isthmus regions a glandular band can be identified, which differentiates the two regions (fig. 53). The egg remains about one hour and fifteen minutes in the isthmus, to form the albumin and the testaceous membrane. The final region of the oviduct is the **uterus**, it is a pouch-like structure where the egg will spend the longer time, about 20 hours approximately, while the shell is formed, pigmented and the cuticle (or bloom) is deposited.

## Study of the head: evaluation of the nasal cavity and the brain

To evaluate the brain, the head is separated by cutting through the atlantooccipital joint. Reflect the skin from the scalp, insert the scissors into the foramen magnum (fig. 54) and cut two parallel longitudinal incisions following the axis of the head and a transversal cut, level with the inner corner of the eye (fig. 55). Then, using tweezers, lift this section of the skull to expose the brain (fig. 56). Remember not to remove the brain from the skull, but to fix it directly in a formalin solution to be able to conduct a histological examination of the brain.

The evaluation of the nasal cavity is performed by a transversal cut across the end section of the beak (fig. 57). The nasal turbinates, infraorbital and lateral orbital sinuses can be seen, and opened along the length to examine the possible presence of exudates (fig. 58a). If the cut is made further towards the cranium, it exposes the nasal vestibule which should not be confused with the sinus (fig. 58b).

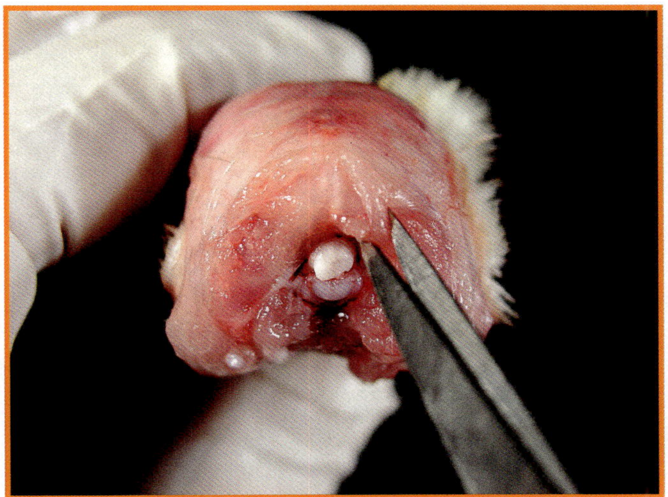

Fig. 54 | Introduce the scissors into the foramen magnum to open the skull.

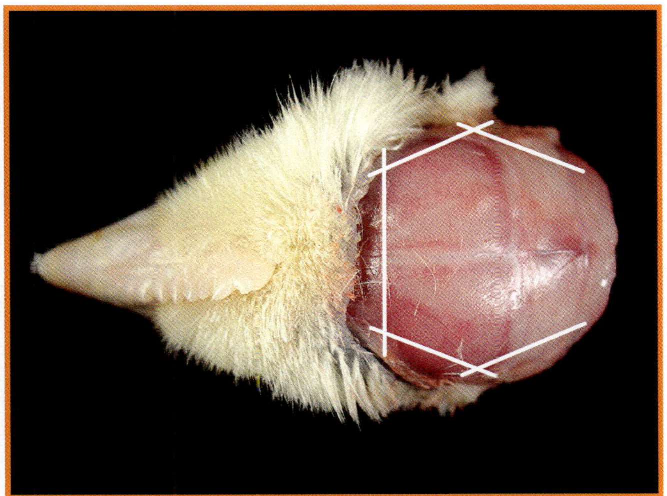

Fig. 55 | Incisions to open the bird's skull and expose the brain.

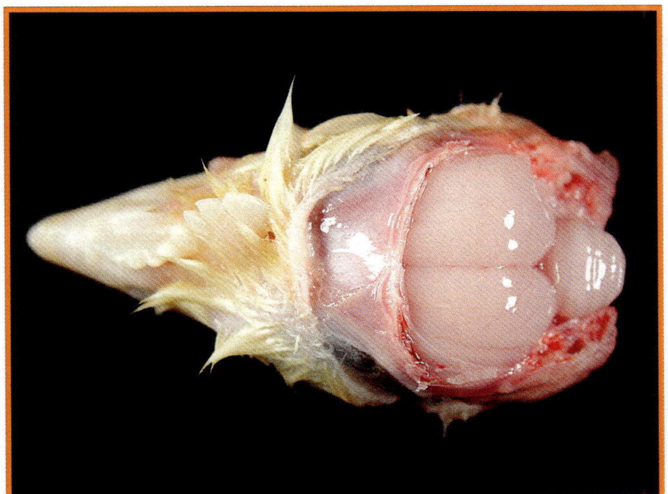

Fig. 56 | Appearance of the brain once the skull is opened.

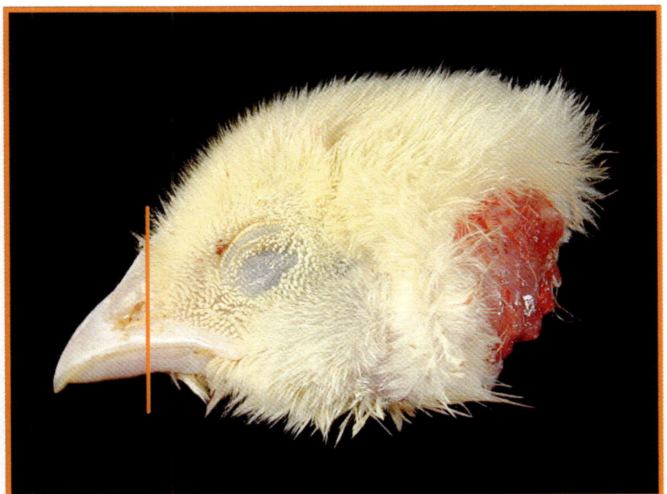

Fig. 57 | Cutting area to visualize the nasal turbinates.

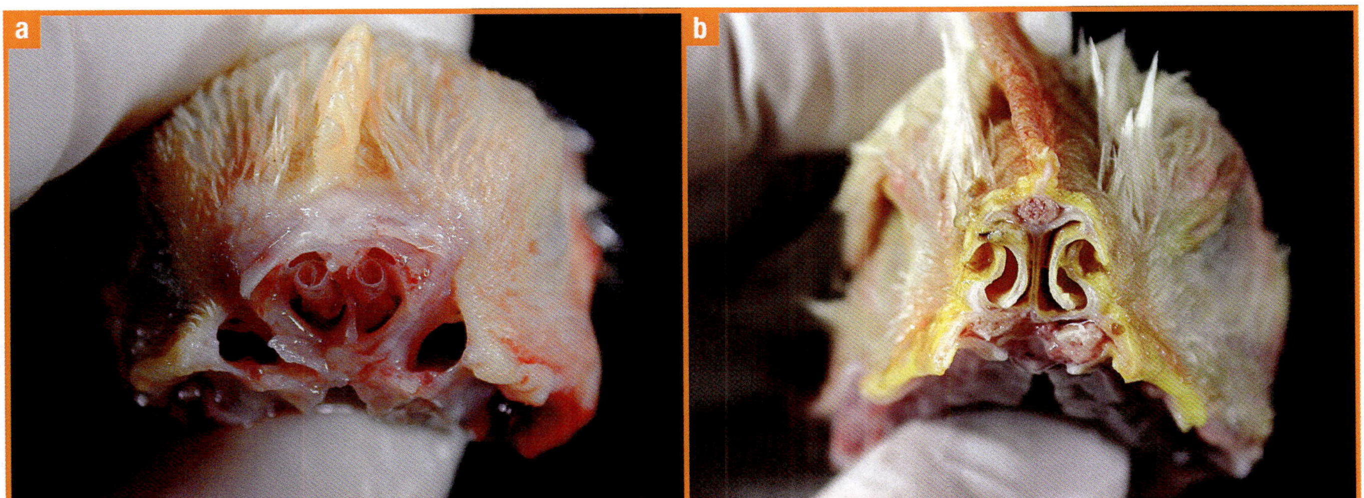

Fig. 58 | Appearance of the nasal cavity with the turbinates and infraorbital sinuses of a healthy bird (a). Appearance of the nasal vestibule in a healthy bird. The turbinates are found caudally (b).

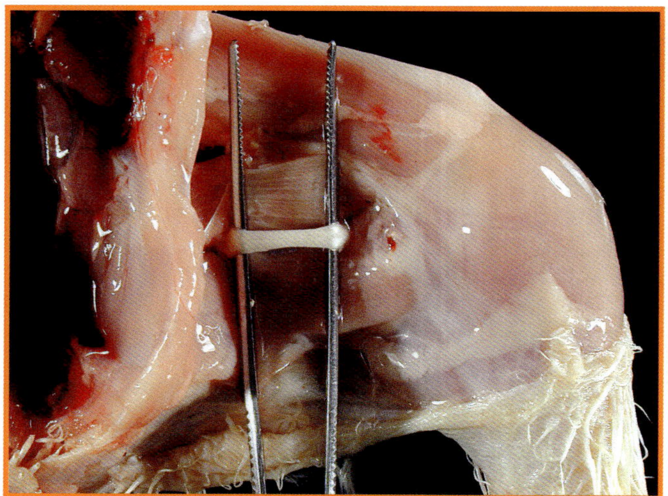

Fig. 59 | Appearance of the sciatic nerve of a healthy bird.

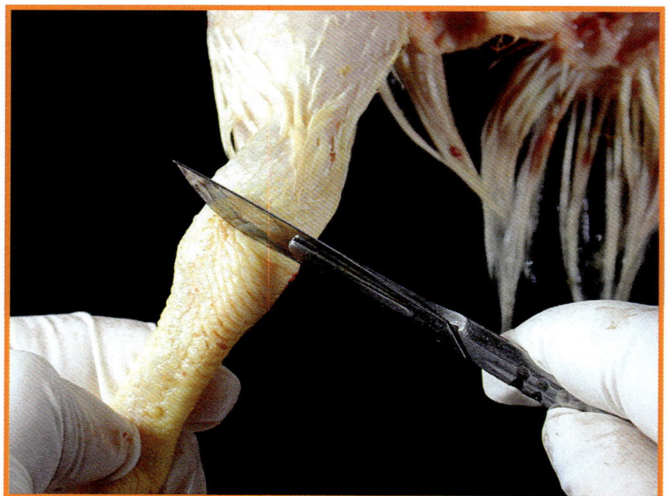

Fig. 60 | Incision with the scalpel to cleanly open the joint.

## Study of the musculoskeletal system: evaluation of the nerves, joints, bones and muscles

Once the sciatic nerves are located below the muscles of the inner thigh, they should be examined. Although the gross evaluation is complicated, it consists of comparing the size of the two nerves to detect swelling. In addition, evaluate the presence of vertical striations (fig. 59).

Also examine the joints, both the femur-tibiotarsal and the tibiotarsal-metatarsal joints. This is achieved by opening the joint with a single cut by a scalpel (fig. 60). The articular cartilage should be smooth and shiny with a small amount of transparent, viscous joint fluid (fig. 61).

The condition of bone mineralisation is found by breaking the tibiotarsus or trying to bend the beak of the animal. In the situation of wanting to examine the presence of lesions of the growth plate, it is necessary to extract a long bone, usually the femur, and open it longitudinally after being decalcified. This same bone serves to take a sample of bone marrow. This is achieved by diagonally fracturing the bone and exposing the bone marrow (fig. 62).

Finally, longitudinal sections of distinct skeletal muscles should be performed, such as the chest, to examine the presence of lesions in the muscles (fig. 63).

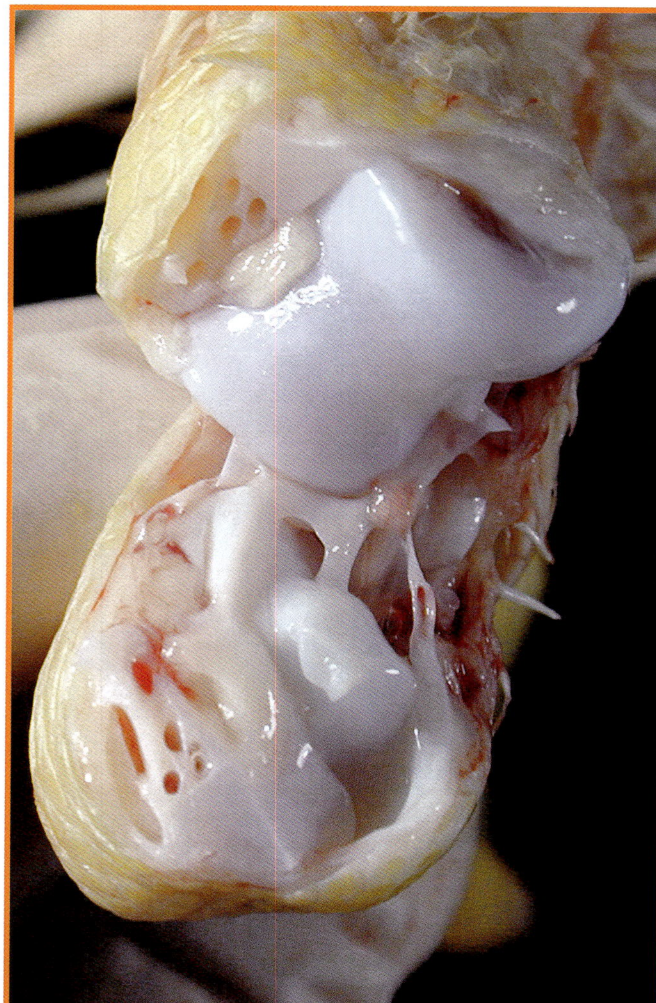

Fig. 61 | Appearance of the joint, opened with only one incision.

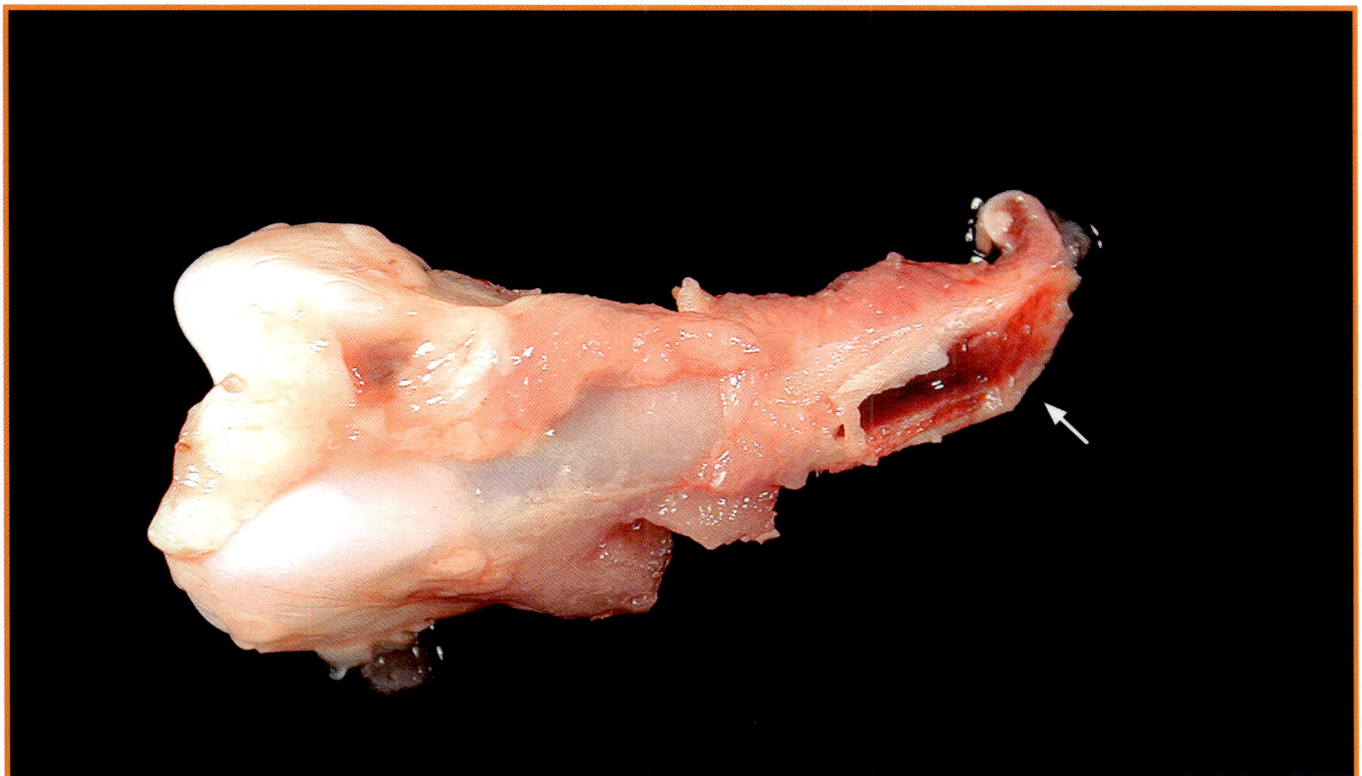

Fig. 62 | Normal appearance of the bone marrow (arrow).

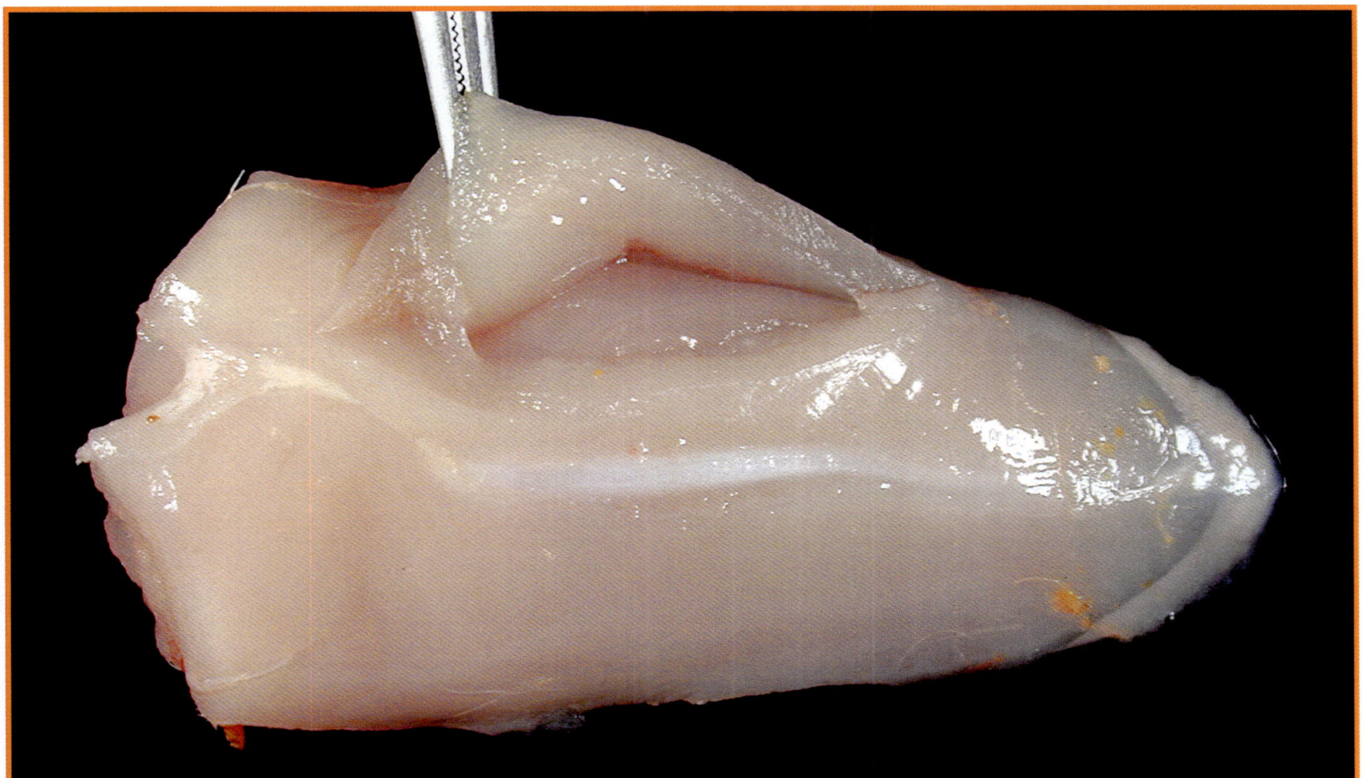

Fig. 63 | Section of the breast muscles to evaluate possible muscular lesions.

CHAPTER 2

# MACROSCOPIC EVALUATION OF THE ORGANS

SKIN AND SUBCUTANEOUS TISSUE

RESPIRATORY SYSTEM

DIGESTIVE SYSTEM AND THE LIVER

CARDIOVASCULAR SYSTEM

LYMPHOHEMATOPOIETIC SYSTEM

GENITOURINARY SYSTEM

MUSCULOSKELETAL SYSTEM

NERVOUS SYSTEM

# Previous aspects to keep in mind

The main objective in performing a necropsy is to evaluate the possible macroscopic lesions of the affected animals. Compiling the gross findings will allow a differential diagnosis to be used to identify the most probable disease and collect the correct samples to confirm it.

The individual examination of each organ or system must also be made in a systematic and orderly way to gather the maximum amount of information possible. This chapter presents an evaluation methodology, as well as the most significant gross lesions of avian organs, apparatus and systems.

# Skin and subcutaneous tissue

The avian integumentary system includes the skin, feathers, and other structures such as the beak, the comb and the wattle. To determine the presence of lesions or alterations in this system, **colour changes, the presence of nodules, scabs or ulcerations, and their distribution** (localised or generalised) should be evaluated. It is worth mentioning that in several cases cutaneous lesions are observed more easily while processing the carcass in the slaughterhouse.

The main lesions that can be observed in the skin and subcutaneous tissue are:

- **Cutaneous haemorrhages:** they may be localised or generalised and of varying sizes, depending on the origin of the lesion. These nonspecific lesions may originate both from a viral infection, for example, avian influenza virus (fig. 1) or infectious anaemia virus (fig. 2) as well as from traumatic causes (fig. 3). They may develop a bluish or greenish colour and even scab formation in the affected regions (fig. 4).
- **Pale skin colour:** a lesion that is observed mainly in the comb or legs and may be secondary to disorders associated with intestinal malabsorption (e. g., coccidiosis) or anaemia.
- **Melanosis:** an observation of dark or black discoloration in the conjunctive tissue or subcutaneous fat (fig. 5). If this discoloration occurs in the subcutaneous tissue of the legs, externally they will appear greenish due to the effect of the mixture of yellow and black (fig. 6). Melanosis has a genetic origin and is caused by a deposit of melanin in abnormal amounts or locations.

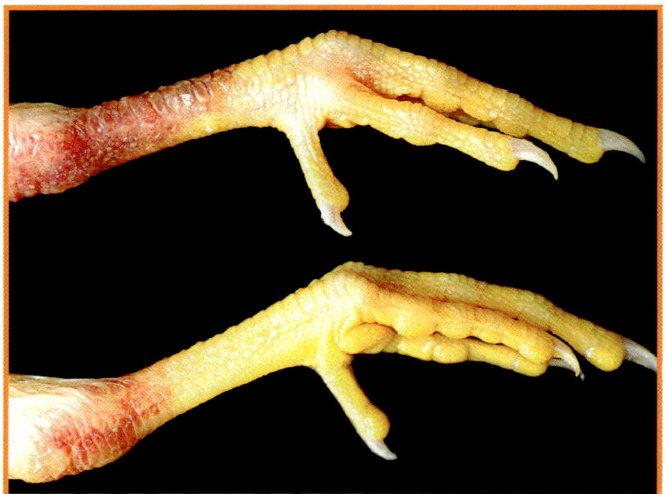

Fig. 1 | Cutaneous haemorrhages in the legs of a bird affected by a highly pathogenic form of avian influenza.

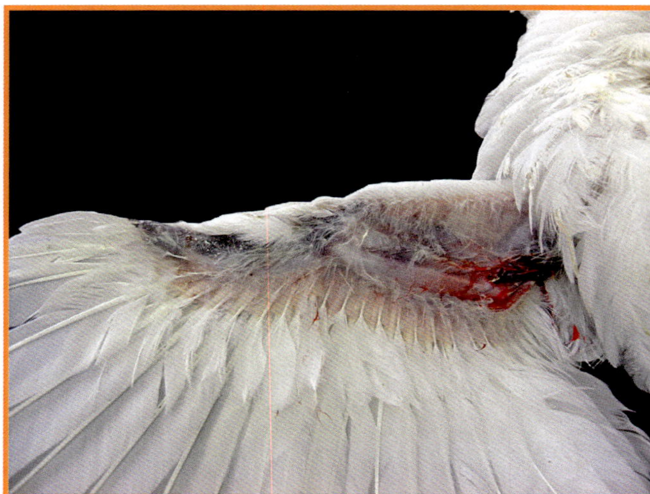

Fig. 2 | Subcutaneous haemorrhages in the wings of a bird affected by avian infectious anaemia.

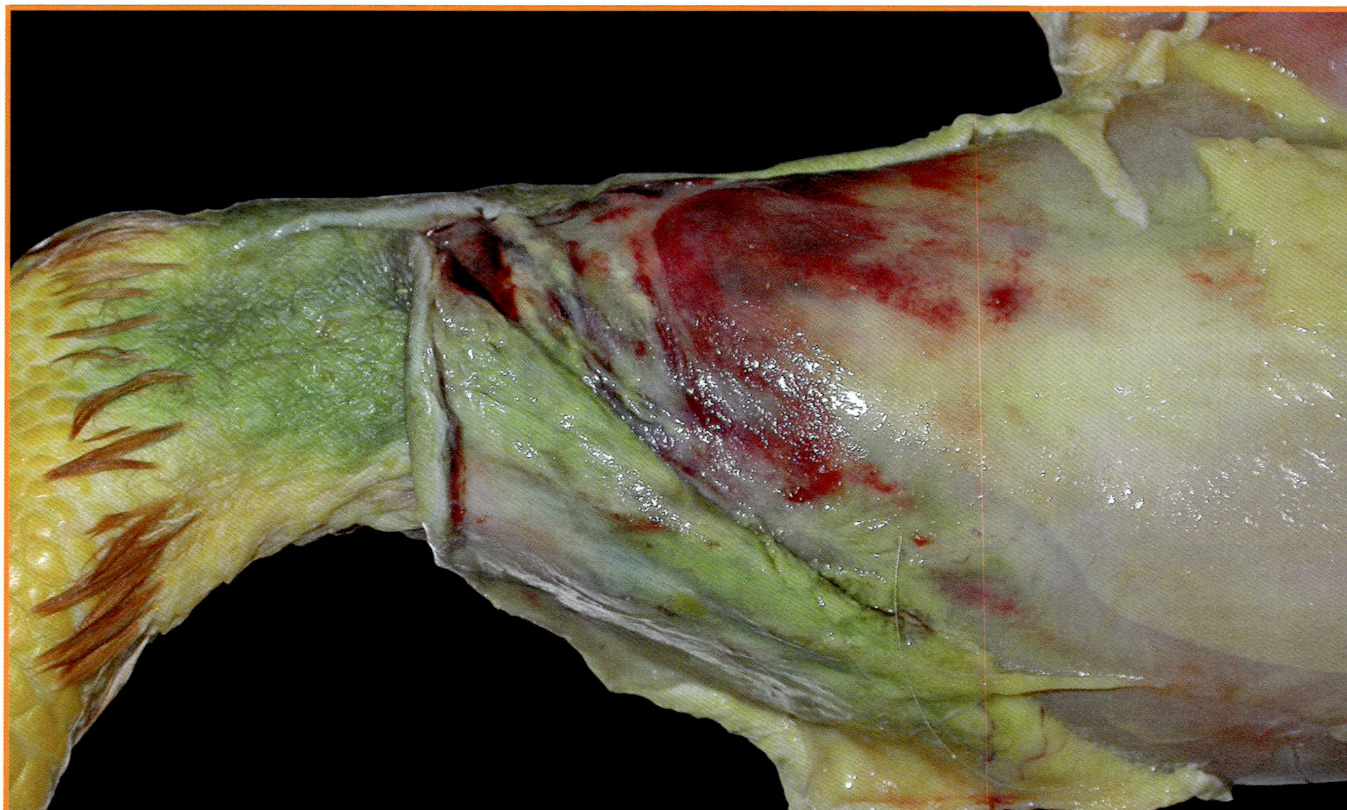

Fig. 3 | Subcutaneous haematoma, possibly of traumatic origin.

- **Dermatitis:** a locally extensive reddened area of the skin associated to cutaneous inflammation with marked oedema and congestion. The causes of dermatitis can be varied, from traumatic problems (abrasion) to bacterial infections, mainly due to *Clostridium* spp. (fig. 7). On occasions, the cutaneous inflammation may be seen with scab formation as in the case of a cutaneous infection associated with the avian pox virus (fig. 8) or with nutritional deficiencies (fig. 9).

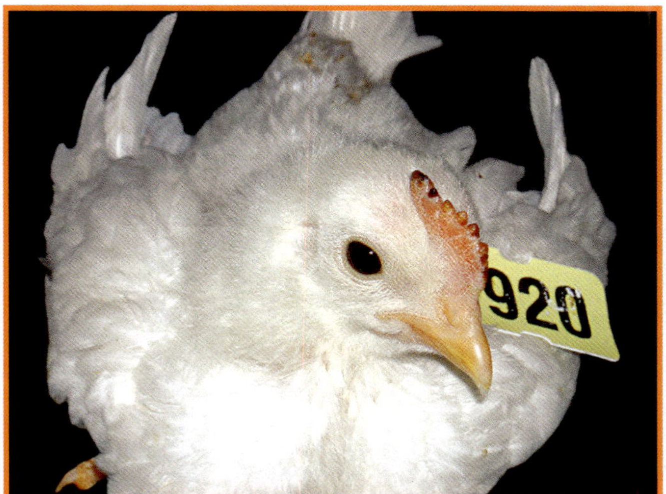


Fig. 4 | Small cyanotic and necrotic areas on the comb of a bird affected by a highly pathogenic form of avian influenza.

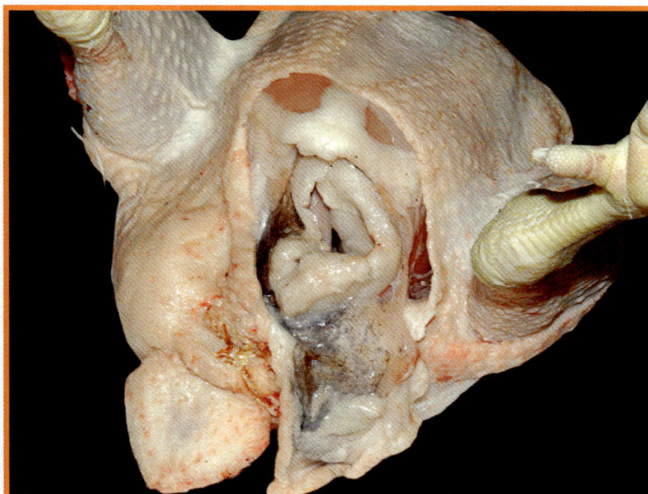

Fig. 5 | Subcutaneous melanosis in the pericloacal area.

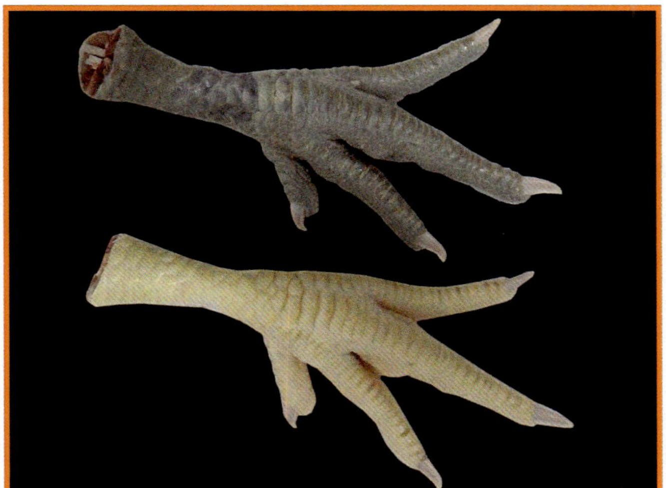

Fig. 6 | Cutaneous melanosis in the legs.

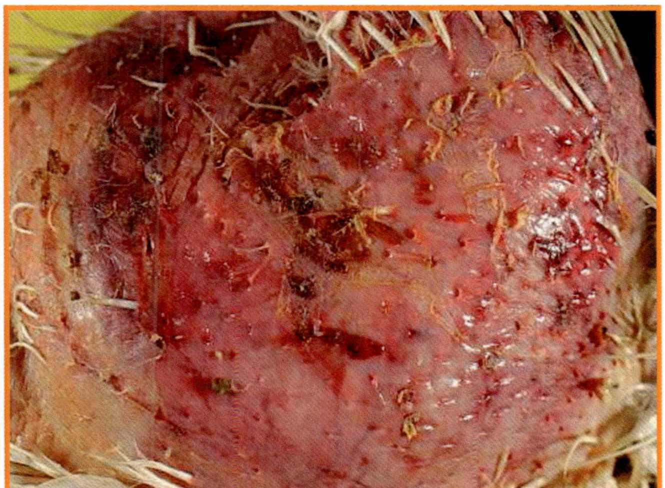

Fig. 7 | Gangrenous dermatitis with marked congestion in the affected area.

- **Omphalitis:** a specific type of dermatitis located in the navel (fig. 10). It is seen in newly hatched chicks and is associated with a local, bacterial infection.
- **Pododermatitis:** a specific type of dermatitis localised on the foot pad and normally associated with a poor quality of bedding/litter. In the first stage, a focal ulceration of the epidermis may be observed (fig. 11) which develops into scab formation or even granulomatous infections of the subcutaneous tissue due to the secondary bacterial contamination (fig. 12).
- **Folliculitis:** a thickening of the feather follicles or the perifollicular region. This lesion is most commonly caused by the Marek's disease virus (fig. 13), although similar gross lesions may be present in bacterial infections or other ne-

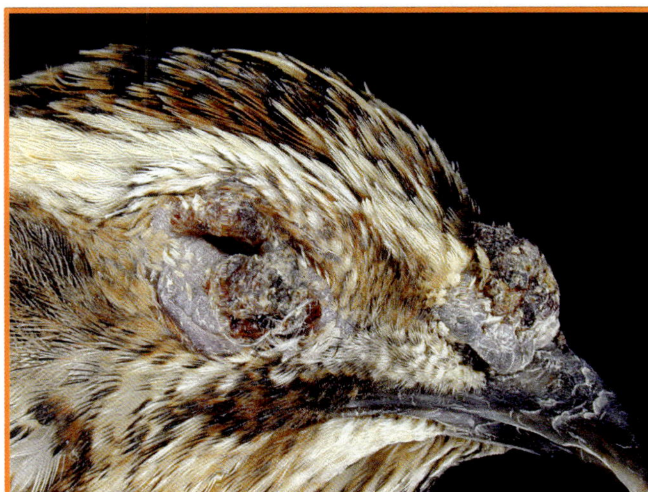

Fig. 8 | Scabby proliferative dermatitis around the eyes and beak of a partridge affected by avian pox.

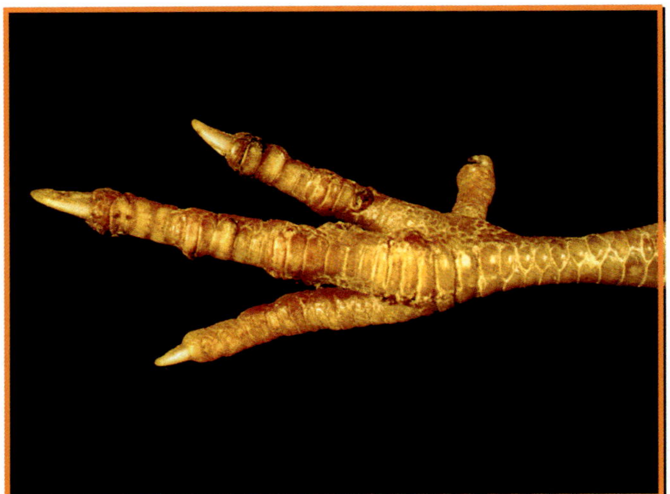

Fig. 9 | A bird's foot displaying dermatitis with scab formation, associated with a pantothenic acid deficiency.

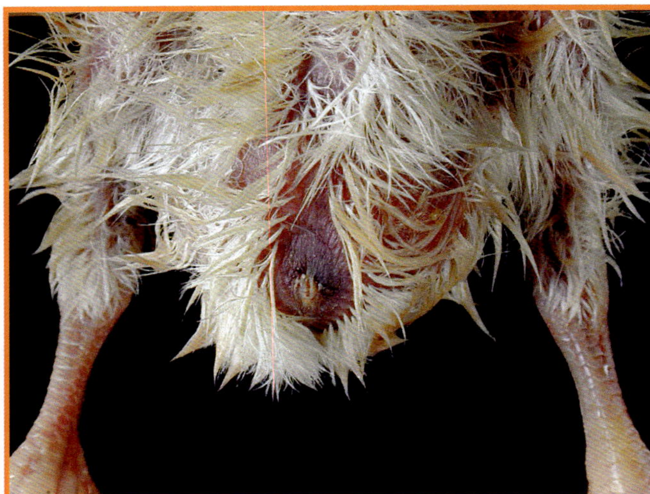

Fig. 10 | Omphalitis in a chick, associated with a bacterial infection.

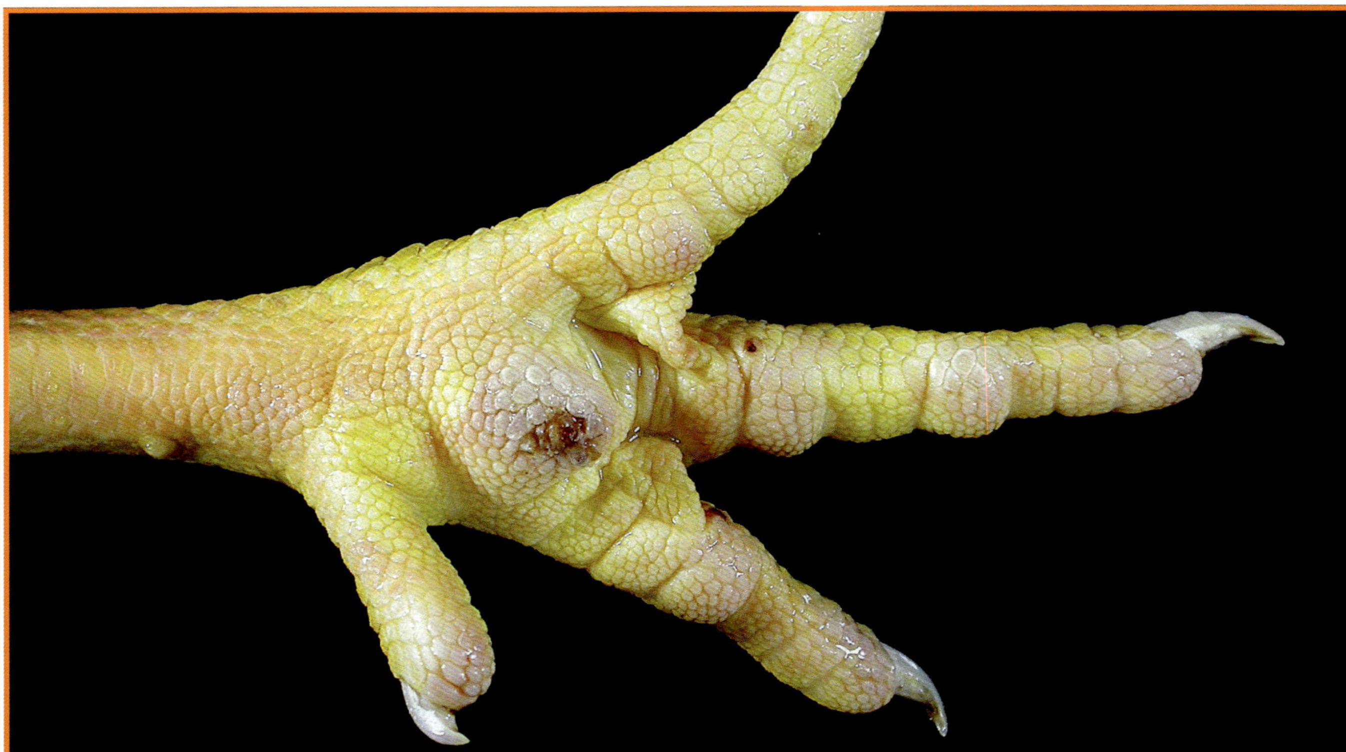

Fig. 11 | Pododermatitis with focal ulceration on the foot pad.

oplastic disorders, such as squamous cell carcinoma. In these cases, the histopathology will determine the source of the lesion.

- **Cellulitis:** there is a thickened affected area externally visible on the carcass, and when cut, the purulent exudate material is yellowish and gelatinous or fibrinocaseous depending on the chronicity of the infection (fig. 14). This lesion is most commonly found around the cloaca, groin and legs, although it can be seen in any area. It is an inflammation of the subcutaneous connective tissue caused by a bacterial infection (various bacteria have been isolated although the most common is *Escherichia coli*).

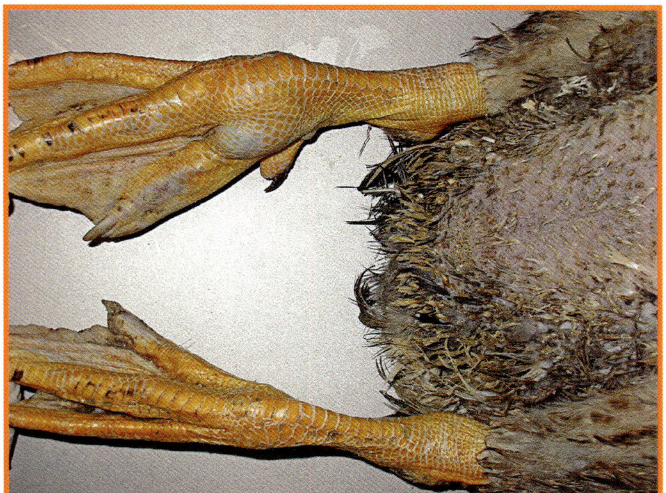

Fig. 12 | Chronic granulomatous pododermatitis in a duck, with thickening of the phalangeal joints.

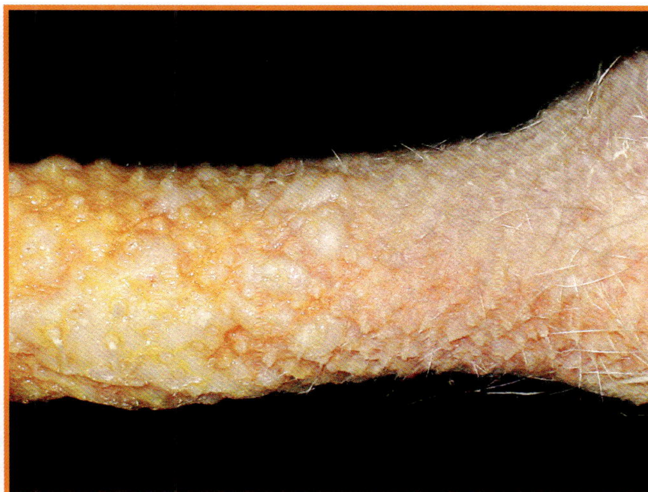

Fig. 13 | Cutanecus lymphoma characterised by perifollicular nodule lesions in the neck region caused by a Marek's disease virus.

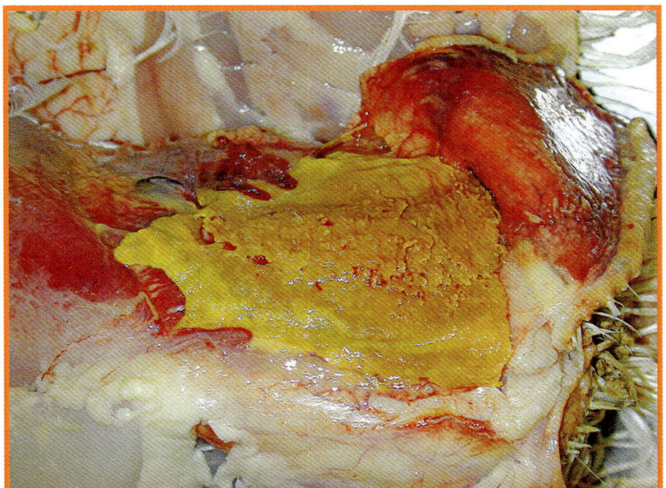

Fig. 14 | Focal fibrinous cellulitis due to *Escherichia coli.*

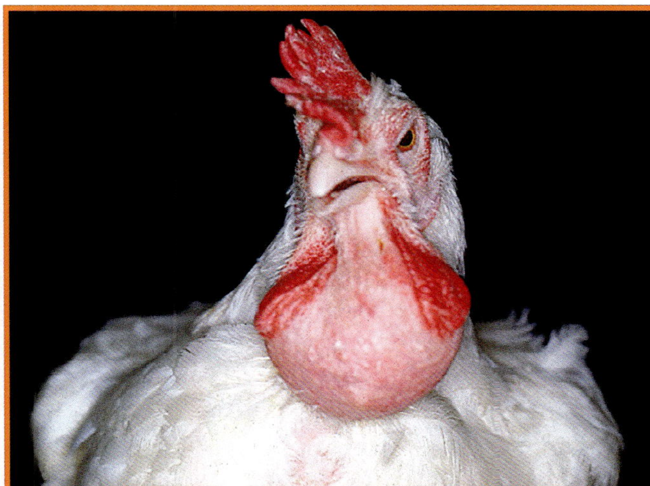

Fig. 15 | Cellulitis in the wattles of a bird affected by avian cholera.

Generally, it is a secondary consequence to a previous injury the animal has suffered or to septicaemia. In *Pasteurella multocida* (avian cholera) infections, cellulitis typically occurs in the wattles which causes the area to become swollen and distended (fig. 15). A yellowish caseous material is found in the interior of the wattles.

- **Sternal cysts:** these lesions are typically observed in the slaughterhouse. Observation shows a cyst formation containing an accumulation of serous exudate within the sternal bursa along the keel bone (fig. 16). This is principally due to the animal being continually prostrated on its keel producing inflammation in this region.

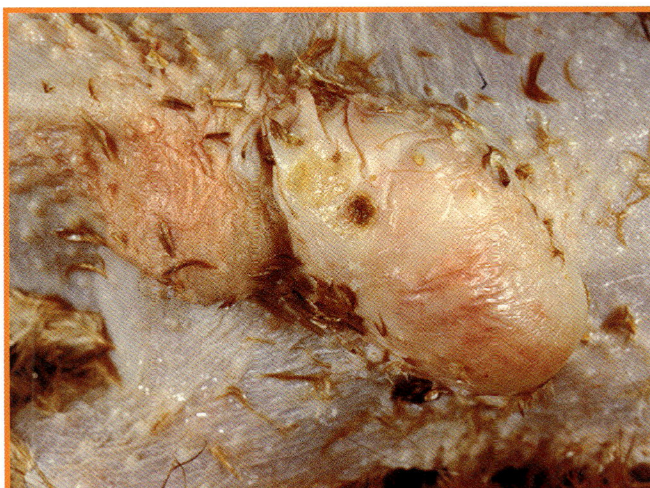

Fig. 16 | Sternal cyst in the subcutaneous tissue of the keel.

# Respiratory system

Respiratory and digestive disorders are probably the main cause of economic losses in poultry production. Avian respiratory ailments are multifactorial disorders in which typically both a primary and secondary causal agents are involved, and once the agents have caused damage to the respiratory system, they proceed to worsen the problem. In general, therefore, the lesions observed are nonspecific or are compatible with more than one disorder or causal agent, and in many cases more than one pathogen is involved. Even so, some lesions may be indicative or suggestive of the involvement of a particular agent.

This section describes the main gross lesions in the different areas of the respiratory system: nasal turbinates, infraorbital sinuses, trachea, lungs and air sacs.

## Nasal turbinates

The evaluation of the nasal turbinates should include their coloration and the presence of exudates. The main disorder observed is rhinitis. This is an inflammation of the nasal turbinates and is characterised by congestion of the mucosa as well as the presence of exudate. The nature of the exudate can help to identify the type of rhinitis, e.g., a mucous exudate is associated with catarrhal rhinitis (fig. 17), and an exudate containing fibrin with fibrinous rhinitis. The most common rhinitis is catarrhal and externally it can be seen by the presence of mucus in the nasal cavities of the birds (figs. 18 and 19). In some cases fibrinous material can also be seen (fig. 20). The swelling of the turbinates may be due to farm environmental factors (dust, ammonia, etc.) as well as to respiratory infection agents such as avian metapneumovirus or avian infectious bronchitis.

## Infraorbital sinuses

The evaluation of the infraorbital sinuses should include observing if the external periorbital area presents swelling or is distended as well as the presence of exudates. The main infraorbital sinus lesion is inflammation or sinusitis. Periorbital swelling is macroscopically observed (fig. 21). Once the sinuses are opened longitudinally, mucous exudate can be observed in the case of catarrhal sinusitis or fibrin in the case of fibrinous sinusitis (fig. 22). The presence of this lesion indicates the involvement of *Mycoplasma* spp., *Avibacterium*

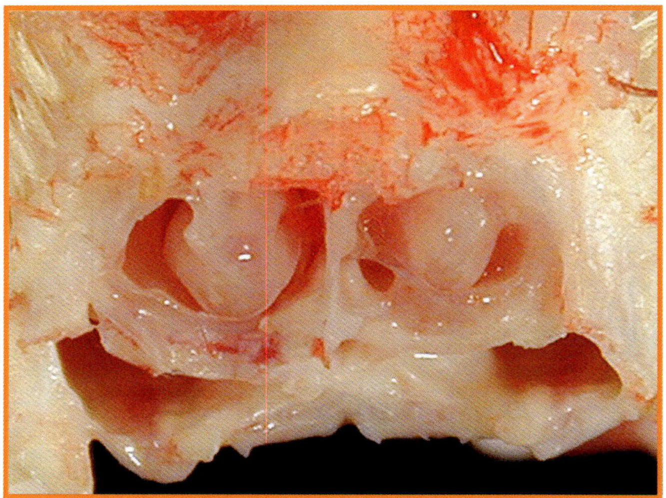

Fig. 17 | Catarrhal rhinitis with mucous exudate in the nasal cavity.

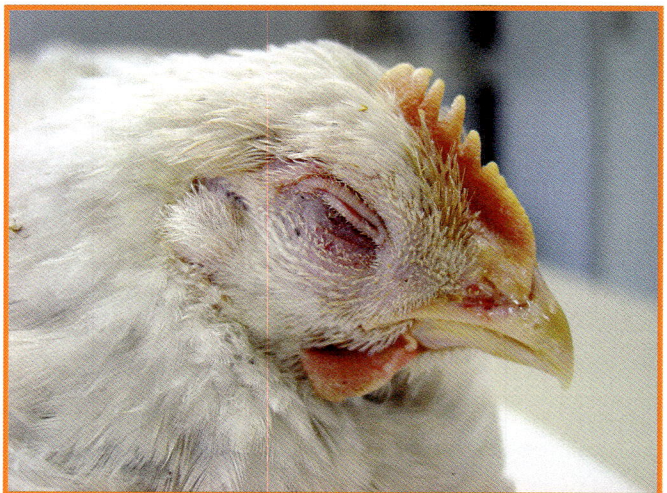

Fig. 18 | Mucous nasal exudate in a bird with a respiratory condition.

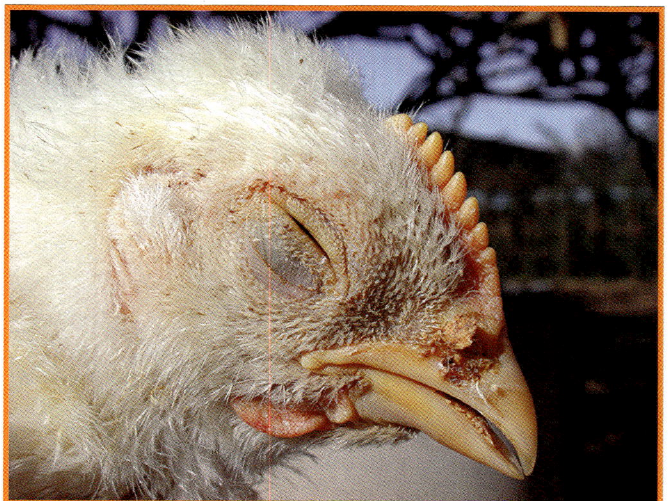

Fig. 19 | Dry mucous nasal exudate in a bird with a respiratory condition.

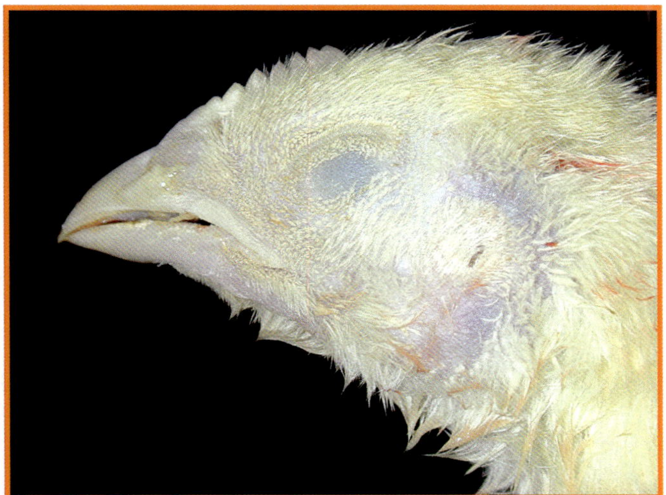

Fig. 20 | Fibrinous nasal exudate in a bird with a respiratory condition.

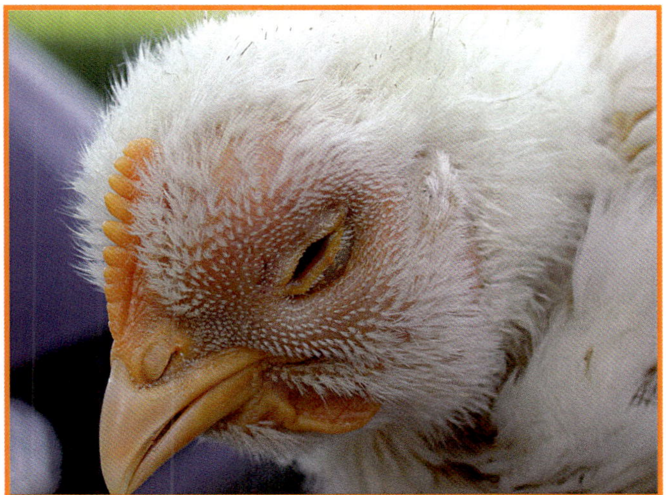

Fig. 21 | Periorbital sinusitis in a chicken. An intense swelling can be seen around the eye.

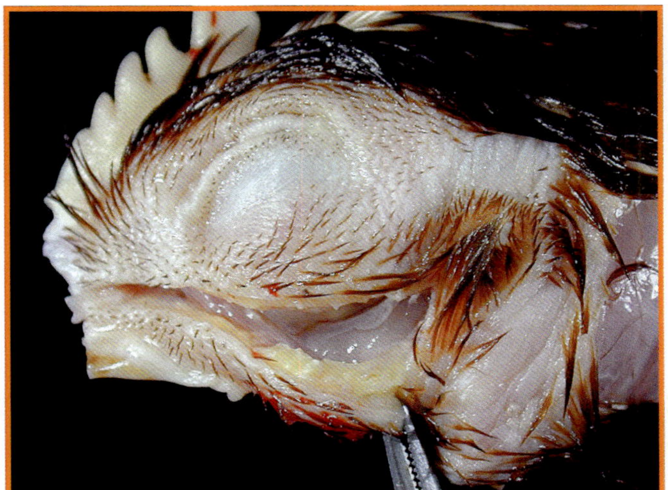

Fig. 22 | Fibrinous infraorbital sinusitis, in a case of avian coryza (an infection by *Avibacterium paragallinarum*).

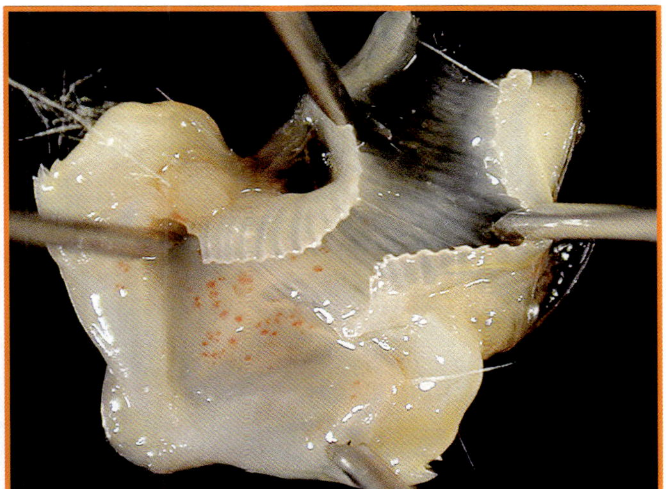

Fig. 23 | Petechiae in the larynx of a bird infected by the avian infectious bronchitis virus.

*paragallinarum* (formerly *Haemophilus paragallinarum*) or avian metapneumovirus (also known as TRT turkey rhinotracheitis), generally with some contaminant in the respiratory condition.

## Trachea

In the trachea the **coloration and aspect** of the tracheal mucus should be examined as well as the **presence of exudates** in the tracheal lumen. The principle lesions are:

- **Petechiae:** petechiae are commonly seen in the laryngeal inlet (fig. 23). In most cases it is caused by irritation due to environmental factors although it can also be caused by a respiratory virus such as infectious bronchitis.
- **Tracheitis:** it is an inflammation of the trachea, characterised by congestion of the mucosa as well as the presence of exudate. Just as in the other regions of the respiratory system, the type of exudate can help with identification:
  - **Catarrhal tracheitis.** In this case there is a mucous exudate (fig. 24). This is probably the most common inflammation, and is associated with respiratory pathogens such as infectious bronchitis virus, avian metapneumovirus, *Mycoplasma* spp. or *Bordetella avium*.

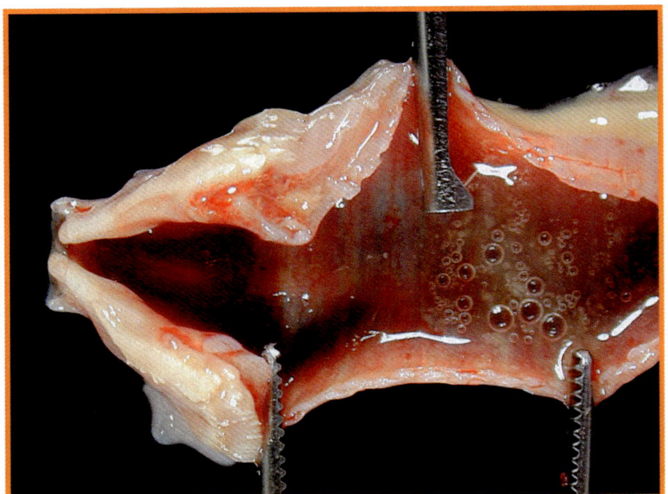
Fig. 24 | Catarrhal tracheitis in a case of avian infectious bronchitis.

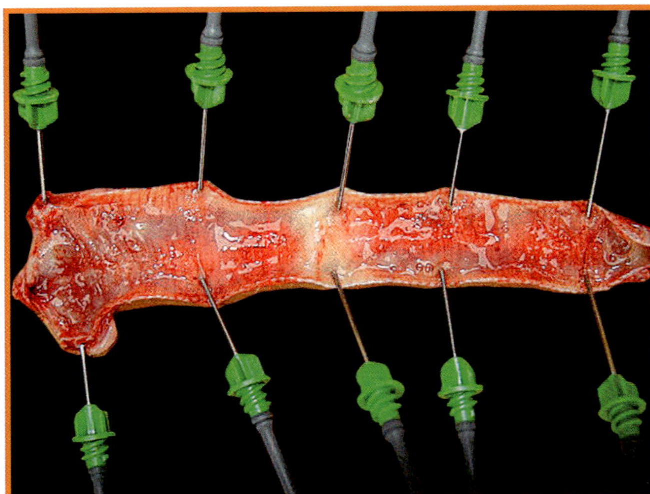
Fig. 25 | Fibrino-necrotic tracheitis in a case of an avian infectious laryngotracheitis virus infection.

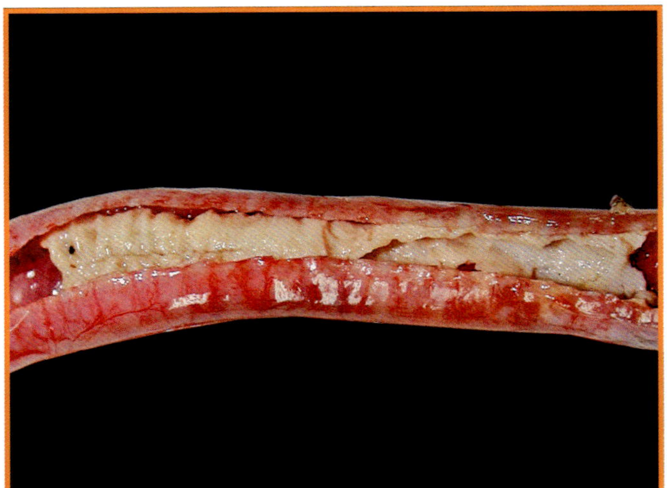
Fig. 26 | Fibrino-necrotic tracheitis in a case of avian pox.

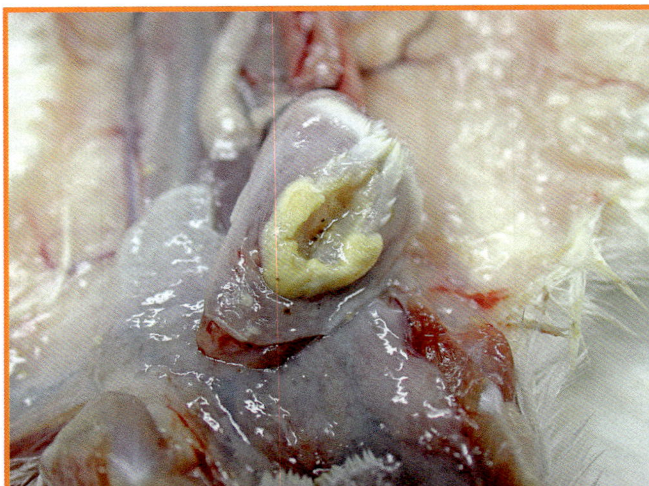
Fig. 27 | Fibrinous exudate in the laryngeal inlet in a case of avian pox.

- **Hemorrhagic tracheitis.** The exudate is hemorrhagic. Although this lesion can be observed in some severe cases of infectious bronchitis, it is usually indicative of more aggressive pathogens such as avian laryngotracheitis virus or Newcastle disease.
- **Fibrino-necrotic tracheitis.** It is characterised by the presence of fibrin or caseous material in the tracheal mucosa (fig. 25). In some cases the fibrin molds into the cylindrical shape of the trachea (fig. 26), or may even cover the laryngeal inlet (fig. 27). This lesion is compatible with the avian pox virus or the avian laryngotracheitis virus. Both diseases can be histologically differentiated, by the presence in the tracheal epithelium of intracytoplasmic inclusion bodies in the pox virus and intranuclear inclusion bodies in the avian infectious laryngotracheitis (figs. 28a and 28b).

## Lungs

Unlike other species, birds' lungs are rather uninformative and very few lesions can be identified macroscopically. Their evaluation should include the coloration, consistency and presence of exudates.

- Congestion: it is characterised by a reddening of the lungs (figs. 29a and 29b). It is a common, but not very specific lesion.

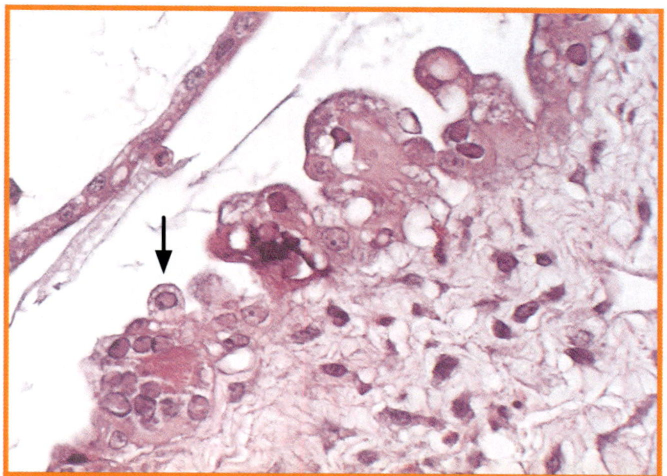

Fig. 28a | Microscopic image of syncytial cells with intranuclear inclusion bodies (arrow) in the tracheal epithelium, in a case of avian infectious laryngotracheitis. H&E stain.

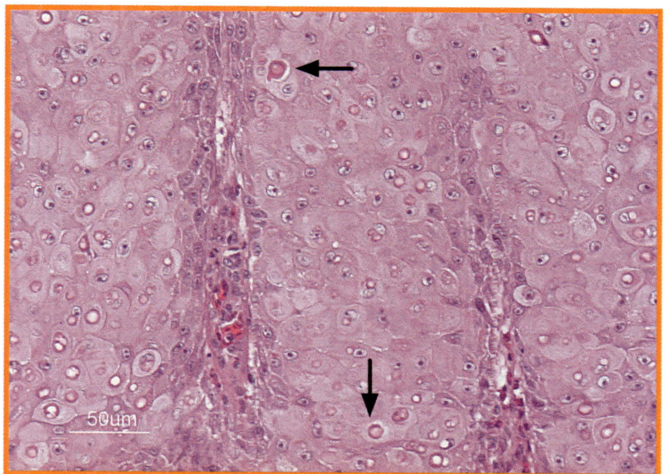


Fig. 28b | A microscopic image of severe hyperplasia of the tracheal epithelium associated with the presence of intracytoplasmic inclusion bodies (arrows) in a case of avian pox virus. H&E stain.

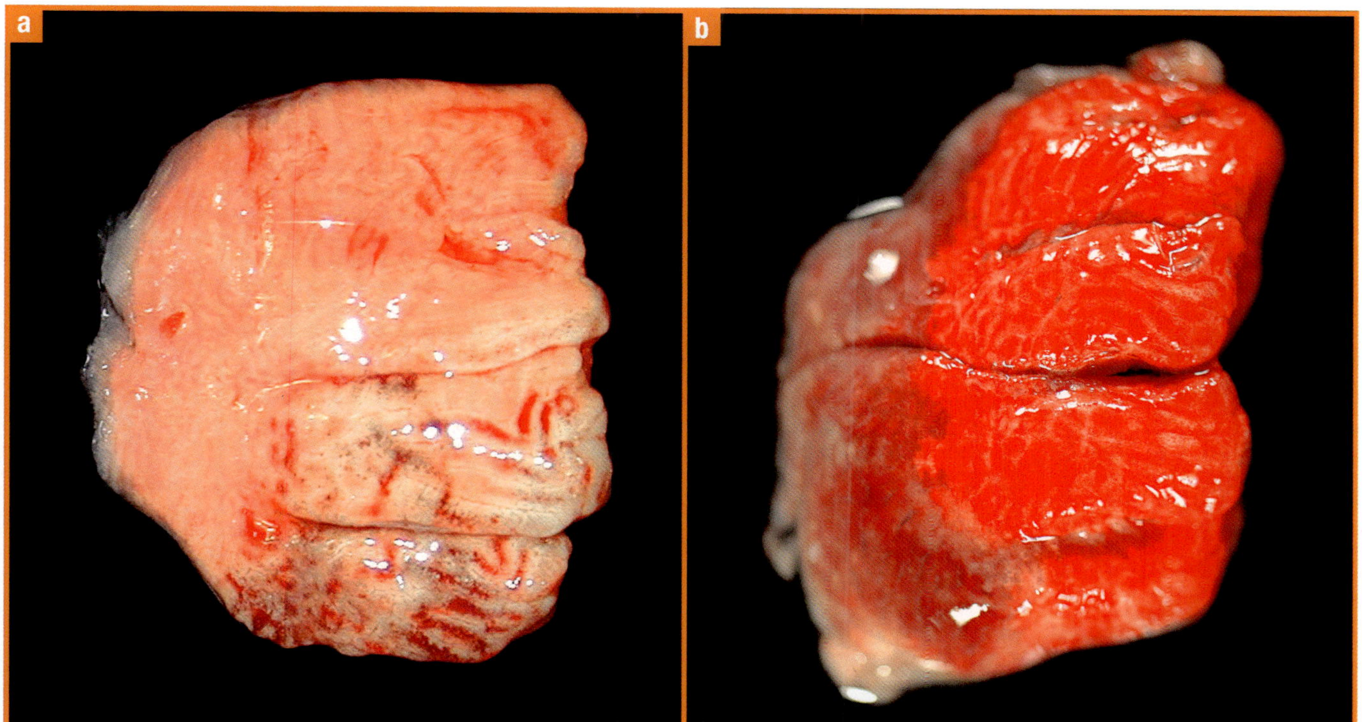


Fig. 29 | Comparison between the appearance of a normal lung (a) and a congestive lung (b).

- **Pneumonia:** it is an inflammation of the lungs. Macroscopically the birds can be distinguished by:
  - **Fibrino-purulent pneumonia.** It is characterised by the presence of fibrin and purulent exudate on the lung surface and in the parabronchi (fig. 30). The examination consists of a cross section to observe the presence of purulent exudate (fig. 31). Also, it is usually accompanied by an increase in lung consistency. This lesion shows the bacterial involvement in respiratory conditions, the most common being: *Escherichia coli, Ornithobacterium rhinotracheale* and *Pasteurella multocida*, especially important in turkeys. Also some septicaemia bacteria can cause this injury, such as *Salmonella typhimurium*. Finally, though more rarely, *Chlamydophila psittaci* may be associated.

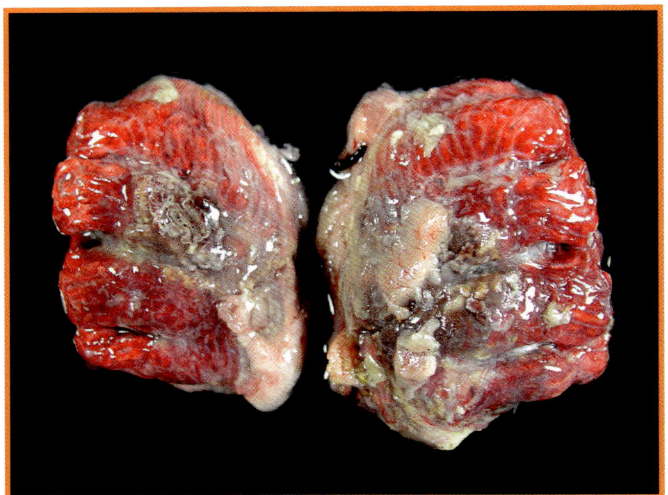

Fig. 30 | Fibrino-purulent pneumonia with fibrinous exudate in the lung parenchyma and on the surface.

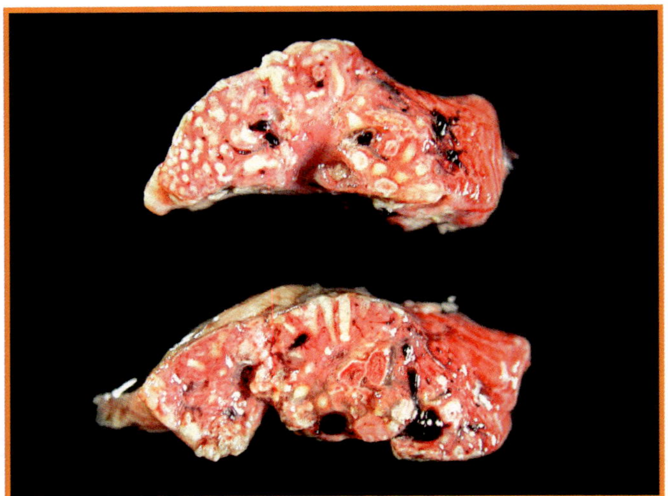

Fig. 31 | Fibrino-purulent pneumonia. A cross section showing fibrino-purulent exudate is seen in the parabronchi.

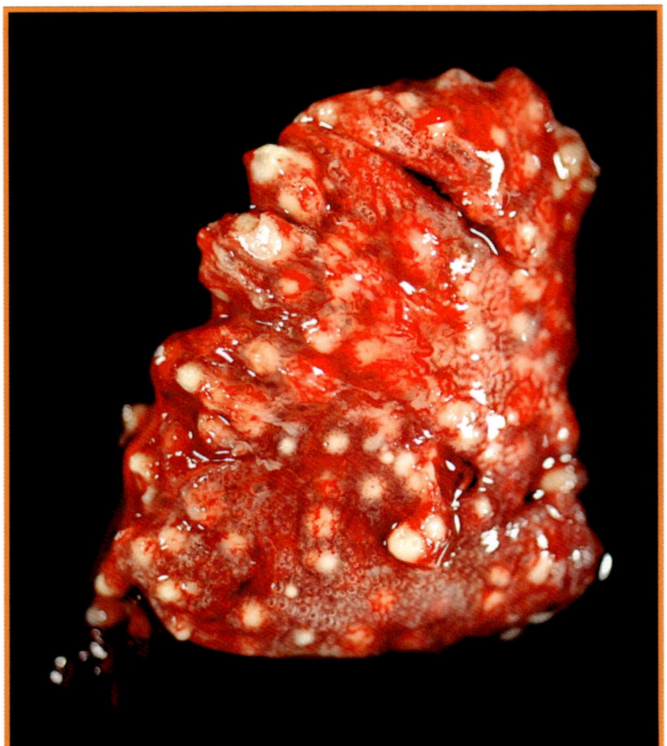

Fig. 32 | Granulomatous pneumonia in a case of pulmonary aspergillosis showing multiple 1-2mm granulomas in the lung parenchyma.

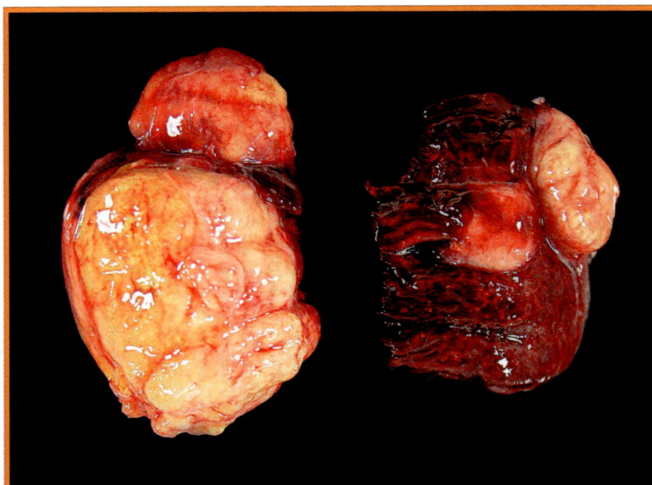

Fig. 33 | Granulomatous pneumonia caused by fungal infection. Multiple large granulomas can be observed on the surface of both lungs.

- **Granulomatous pneumonia.** The presence of small nodules or granulomas can be grossly seen in the lung parenchyma (figs. 32 and 33). They can be confused with tumours, therefore, a tissue histology is necessary. Two main causes are associated with granulomatous pneumonia. The most common is fungal infection mostly associated with *Aspergillus* spp., although other fungi such as *Ochroconis gallopavum* (formerly known as *Dactylaria gallopava*) or zygomycetes can also cause these lesions (figs. 34a and 34b). Although less common today, granulomatous pneumonia is also characteristic of tuberculosis. In all cases, histopathology will differentiate the causes.
- Tumours: observation of the presence of nodules in the lung parenchyma can be confused with granulomatous pneumonia (fig. 35). They are not very common, and may be primary or metastatic tumours, although the most frequent are pulmonary lymphomas caused by Marek's disease.

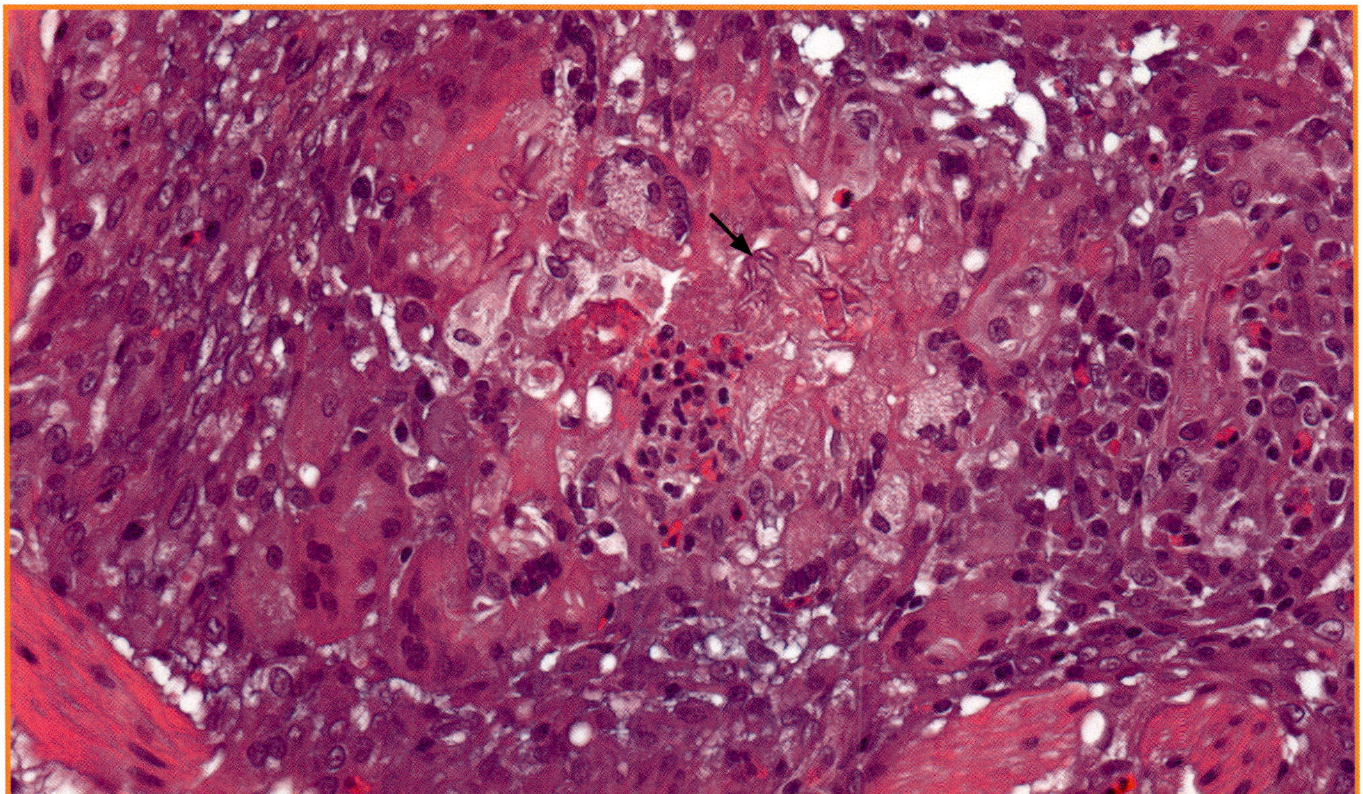

Fig. 34a | Microscopic image of a fungal granuloma. Remains of necrotic material and fungal forms surrounded by multinucleated giant cells can be seen in the centre (arrow). H&E stain.

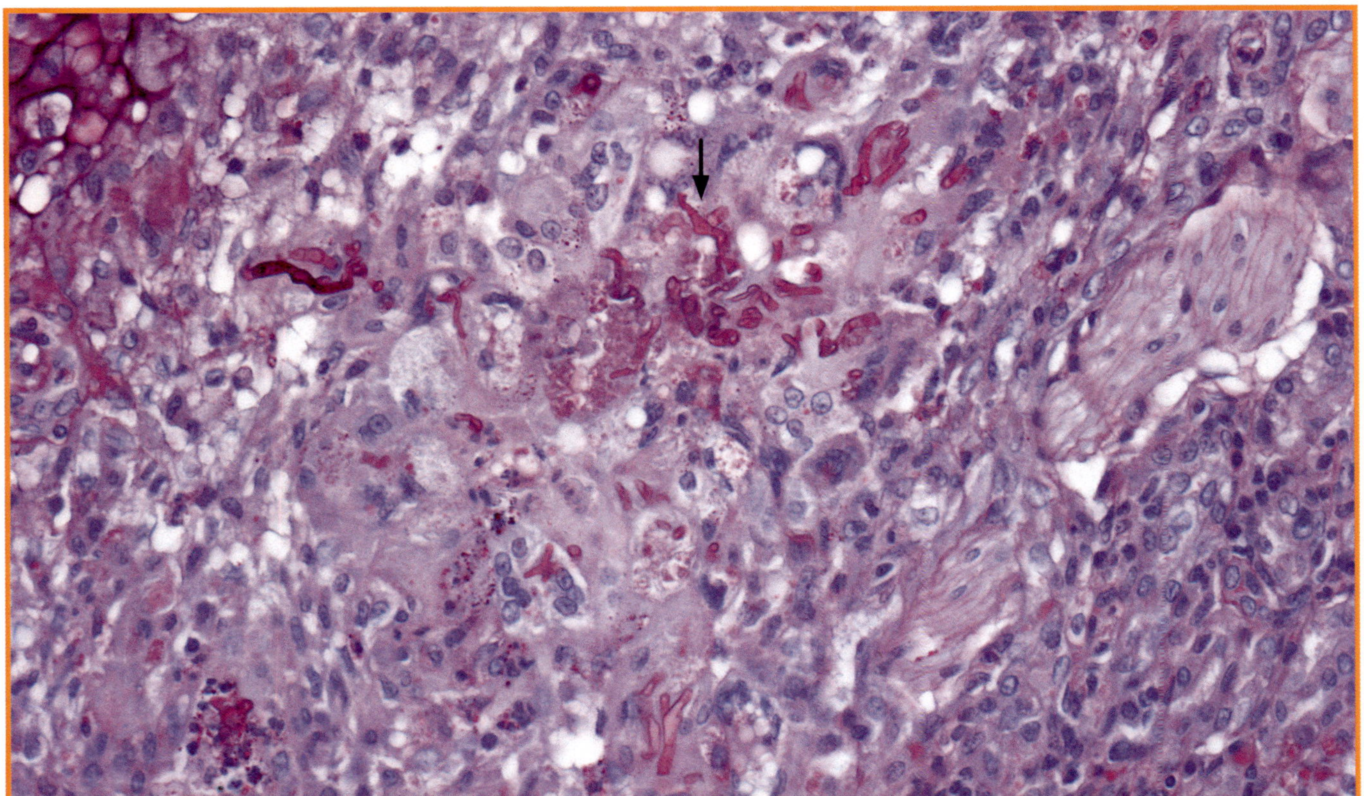

Fig. 34b | Microscopic image of a fungal granuloma using special stains, which differentiates the morphology of the zygomycete hyphae (arrow). PAS stain.

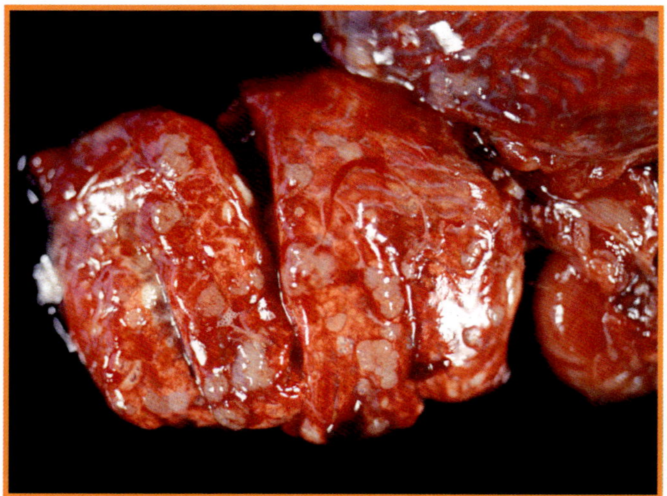
Fig. 35 | Lung adenocarcinoma.

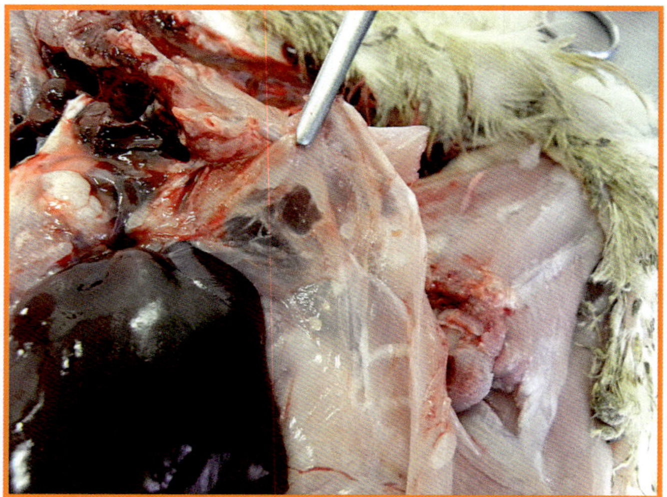
Fig. 36 | Fibrinous airsacculitis with turbidity of the air sacs.

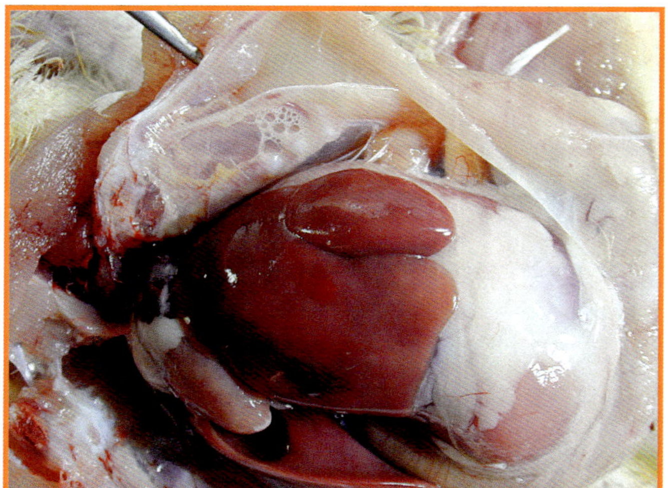
Fig. 37 | Fibrinous airsacculitis in a case of mycoplasmosis.

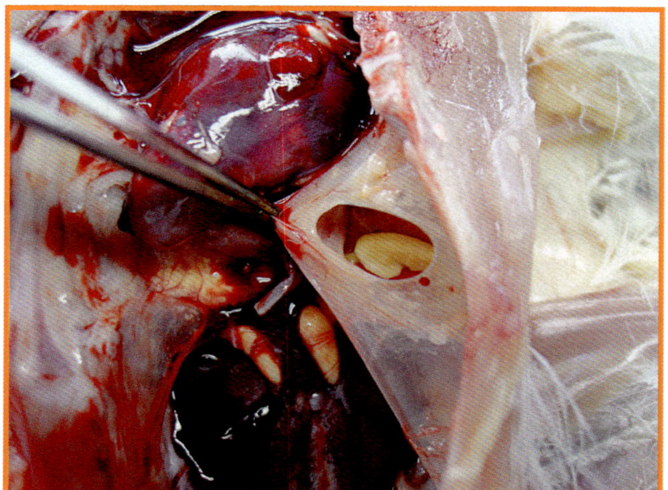
Fig. 38 | Fibrinous airsacculitis in a case of mycoplasmosis.

## Air sacs

Evaluation of the air sacs includes observing the opacity, the presence of exudates in the lumen, and/or the presence of nodules on the surface. The primary lesion is inflammation or airsacculitis.

- Fibrinous airsacculitis: in the initial stages it is characterised by opacity or turbidity of the air sacs (fig. 36). Later, froth and fibrin may be observed in the interior of the air sacs (figs. 37 and 38). In all cases, bacteria are involved with the most common being *Mycoplasma* spp., *Escherichia coli* and *Pasteurella multocida*.
- Granulomatous airsacculitis: in this case, nodules, granulomas or plaques can be observed on the air sac surface (fig. 39) which are associated primarily with fungal infections.

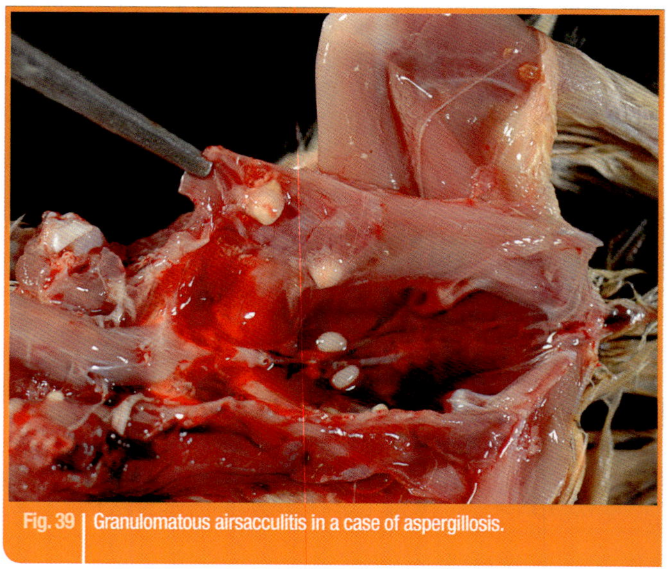
Fig. 39 | Granulomatous airsacculitis in a case of aspergillosis.

# Digestive system

Avian digestive disorders have a direct (mortality) and indirect (lower conversion rate) consequence on batch productivity. In addition, they affect both batch homogeneity producing inequality, and the quality of the carcass, as the conditions of the bedding or litter usually deteriorate. Despite this, gross lesions in the avian digestive tract, especially changes in the intestinal contents, are neither pathognomonic nor very indicative of the causative agent in most cases.

This section describes the main macroscopic lesions of the different areas of the digestive system: oral cavity, oesophagus, proventriculus, gizzard, intestine, pancreas and liver.

## Oral cavity

The evaluation of the oral cavity should include its coloration and the presence of ulcerations, proliferative lesions and exudates. The most common pathological alterations in the oral cavity are inflammation or stomatitis:

- Ulcerative or fibrino-necrotic stomatitis: it is characterised by the presence of ulcers or erosions normally covered by fibrin in the oral mucosa (fig. 40). It is mainly associated with contact with chemical or caustic substances (quaternary ammonium or copper sulphate) or the result of mycotoxins (trichothecenes).
- Proliferative stomatitis: it consists of oral epithelium which often ulcerates (fig. 41). It is mainly associated with avian pox, trichomoniasis and candidiasis.

## Oesophagus and crop

Just as in the oral cavity, the evaluation of the oesophagus and the crop should include their coloration, the presence of ulcerations and the presence of exudates. The most common pathological alterations in these organs are:

- Dilation of the crop: an enlargement of the crop and a thinning of the crop wall is observed (figs. 42 and 43). It is usually a sporadic problem and is related to excessive water consumption, nervous paralysis, or impacted contents.
- Squamous metaplasia: it is characterised by the presence of thickened areas in the mucosa of the oesophagus where the mucosal epithelium has been replaced by keratinized squamous epithelium. Usually associated with a vitamin A deficiency.

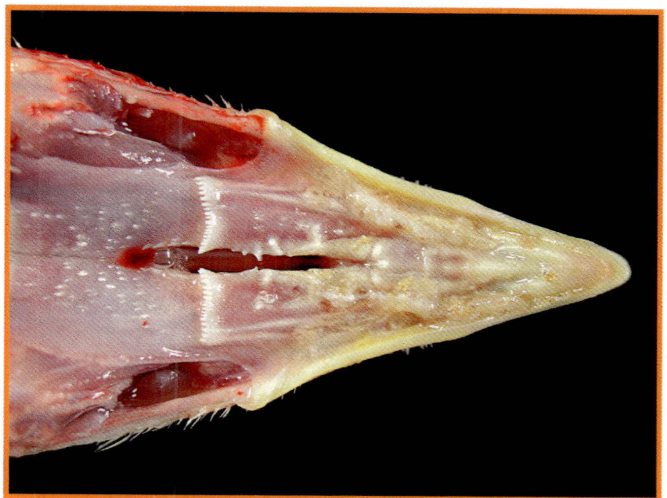

Fig. 40 | Fibrino-necrotic stomatitis with fibrin on the surface of the palate.

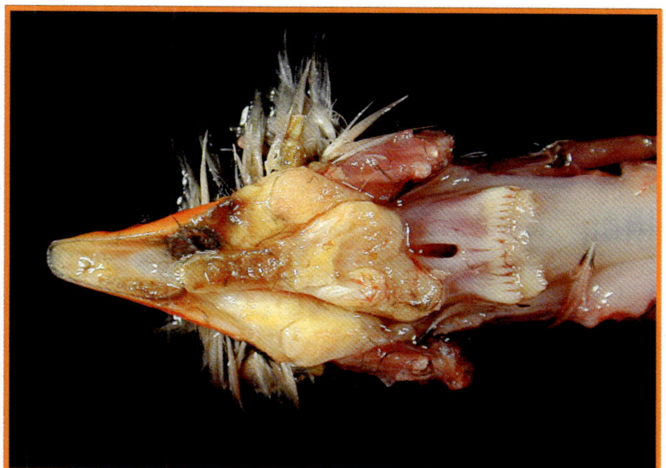

Fig. 41 | Proliferative stomatitis in a partridge affected by avian pox. Thickening of the oral mucosa and the presence of fibrin on the surface can be seen.

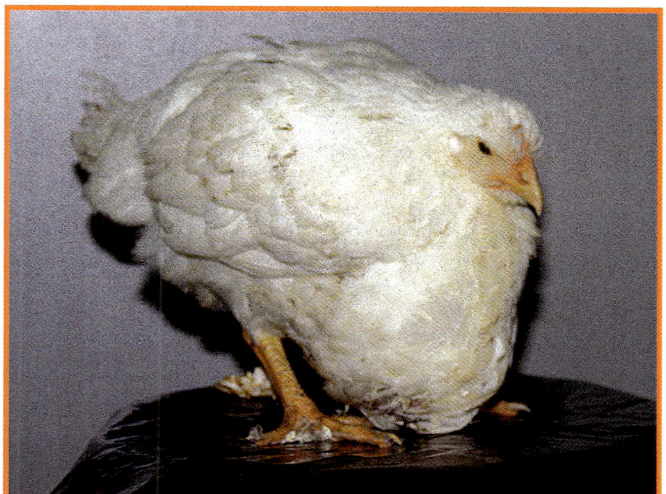

Fig. 42 | Dilation of the crop in a broiler chicken.

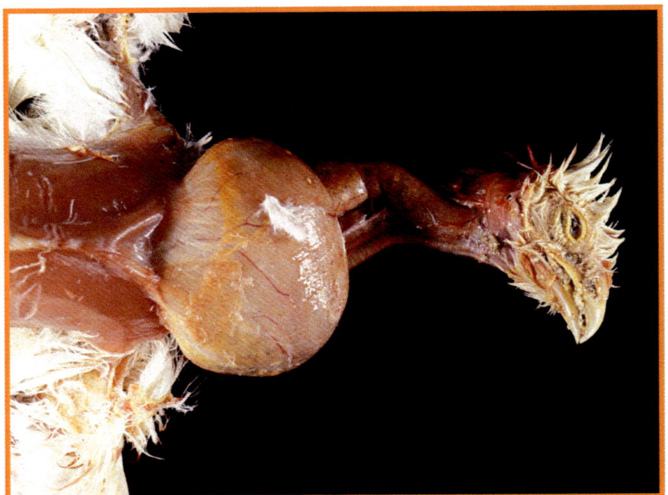

Fig. 43 | Dilation of the crop in a broiler chicken.

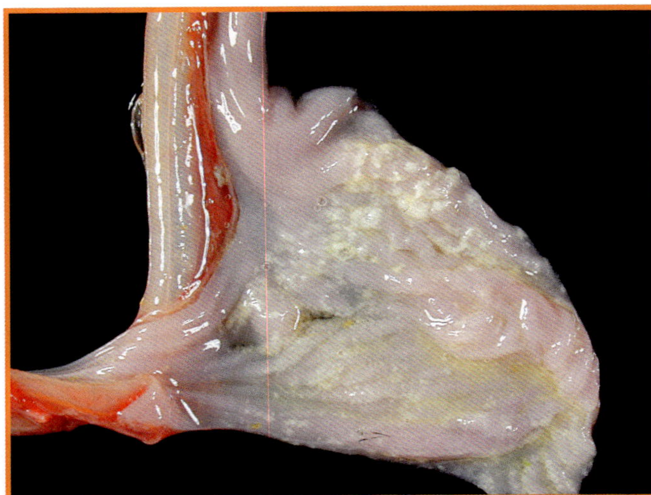

Fig. 44 | Proliferative ingluvitis in a case of candidiasis.

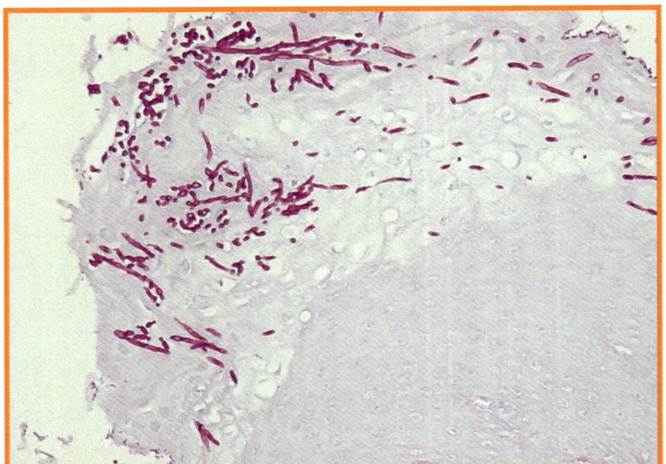

Fig. 45 | Microscopic image in which a proliferation of the crop mucosa and the presence of fungal forms, consistent with *Candida albicans*, penetrate the mucosa. PAS stain.

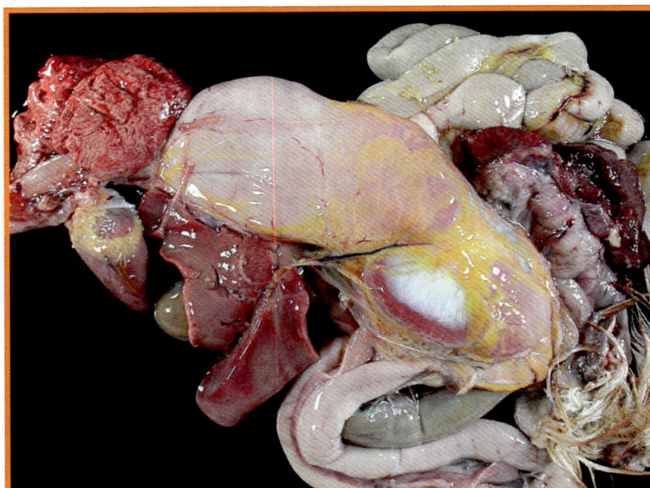

Fig. 46 | Proventricular dilatation in a broiler.

- **Inflammation:** the inflamation of the oesophagus is known as oesophagitis and the inflamation of the crop is known as ingluvitis. Observation shows the wall thickened and the presence of white areas on the mucosa (fig. 44). The main causes are infection by *Candida albicans* (fig. 45) or *Trichomonas gallinae*.

## Proventriculus

The evaluation of the proventriculus should include the **coloration of the mucosa**, the **thickness of the proventriculum wall** and the **appearance of the glands**. Below are the most common pathological alterations in the proventriculus:

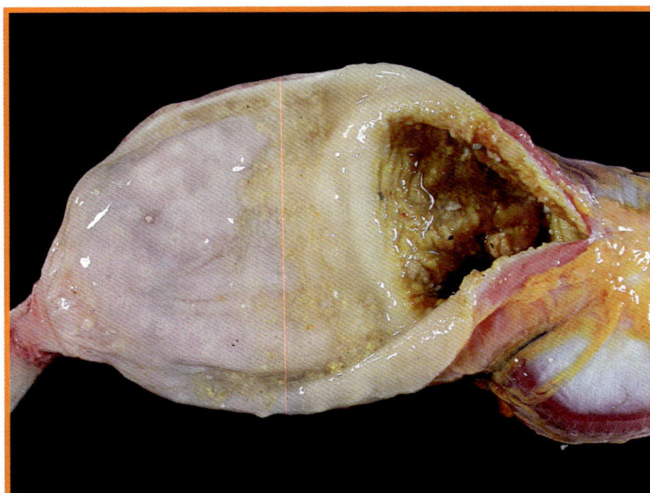

Fig. 47 | Proventricular dilatation. A thinning of the proventricular wall can be seen at the opening.

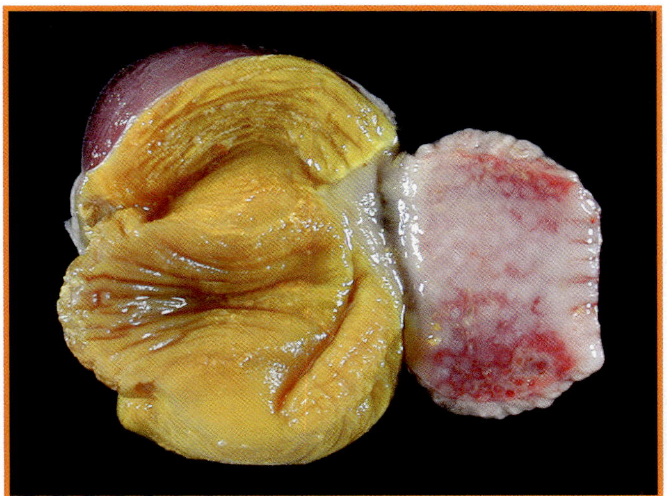

Fig. 48 | Generalised haemorrhages in the proventriculus mucosa IBD (Gumboro disease).

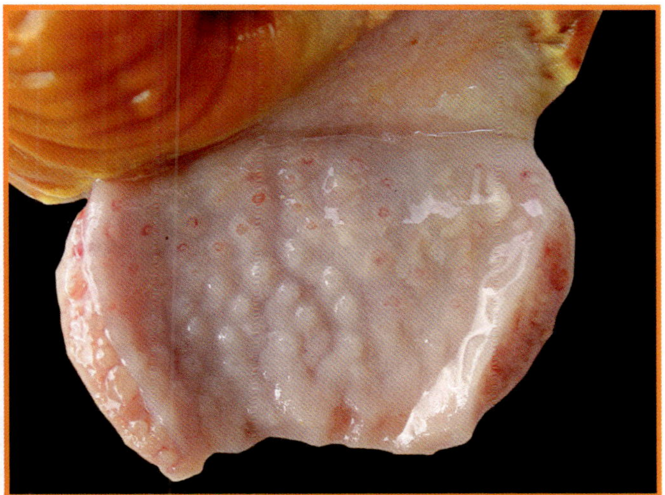

Fig. 49 | Haemorrages around the proventricular glands.

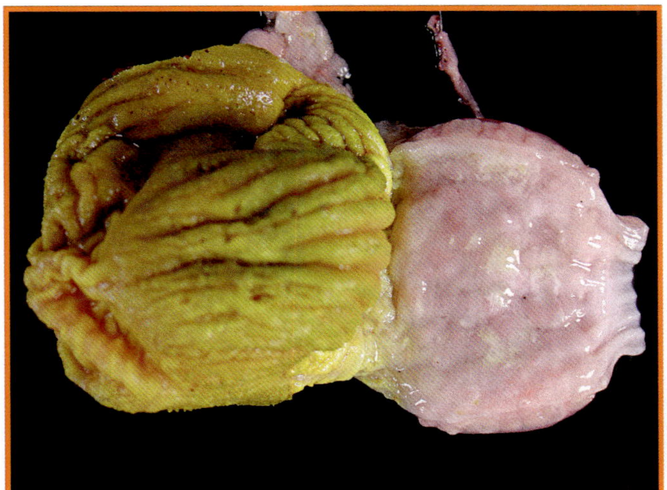

Fig. 50 | Proventriculitis with marked increase in the proventricular wall thickness in a case of transmissible viral proventriculitis.

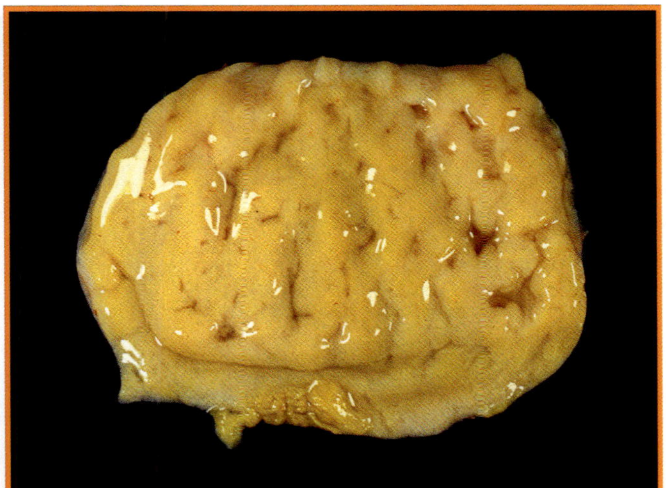

Fig. 51 | Proventricular lymphoma with thickening of the wall and of the proventricular glands in a case of avian leukosis.

- **Dilation:** an enlarged proventriculus is seen (fig. 46) and once it is opened a thinning of the wall is observed (fig. 47). It is usually a sporadic problem, although it has been related to a reovirus infection (malabsorption syndrome).
- **Haemorrhages:** they may be diffuse (fig. 48) or localised around the glands (fig. 49). They may be associated with viral infections such as IBD (Gumboro disease) or Newcastle disease although they may also be a nonspecific alteration.
- **Proventriculitis:** it is an inflammation of the proventriculus. The most obvious gross change is the thickening of the proventricular wall, in some cases accompanied by gland dilation as seen in the cross section of the proventricular wall (fig. 50). In many cases the lesion is nonspecific. It may be associated with diet (enzymes or type of diet), viral infections (adenovirus or Newcastle virus) or to mycotoxins.
- **Tumours:** the most common is lymphoma due to Marek's disease virus or avian leukosis (fig. 51). The macroscopic image shows thickening of the wall and gland dilation, very similar to proventriculitis.

## Gizzard

The evaluation of the gizzard includes the **appearance and presence of ulcerations** in the coilin layer, and the **appearance of the mucosa** once it is separated from the

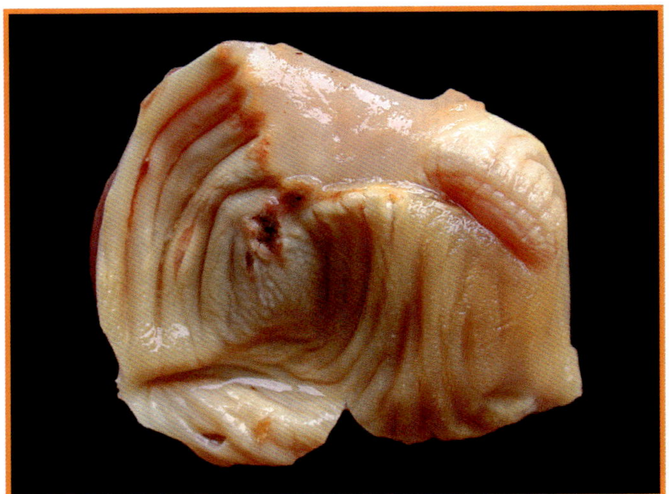

Fig. 52 | Focal ulcerative ventriculitis.

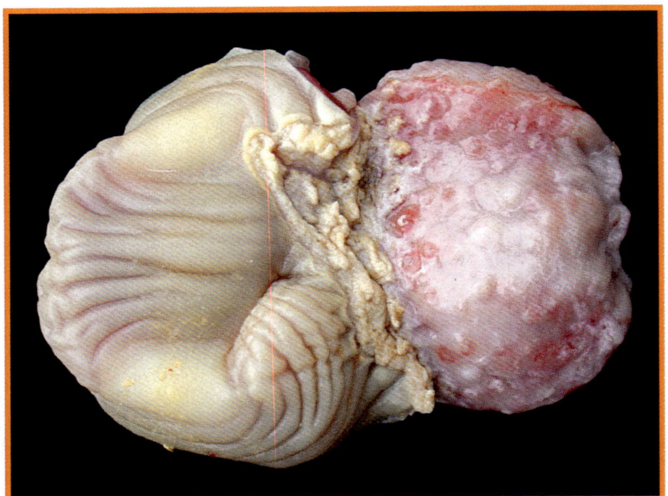

Fig. 53 | Focally extensive ulcerative ventriculitis at the entrance of the gizzard.

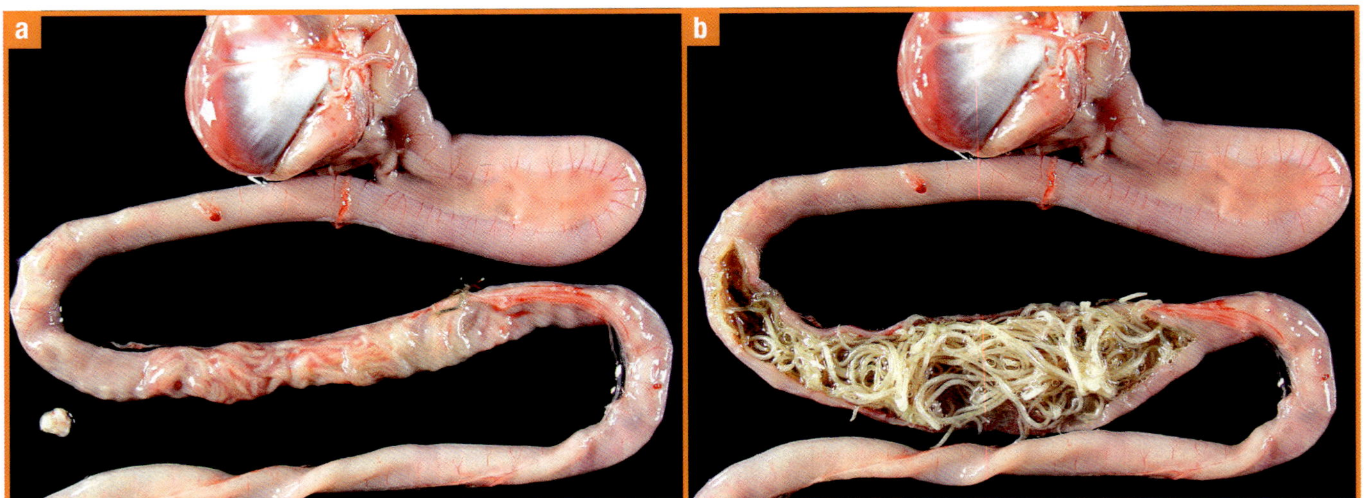

Fig. 54 | Intestinal obstruction from massive parasitisation. A dilated intestinal loop section can be seen (a). A longitudinal section of the obstructed segment where there is the massive presence of parasitic nematodes (b).

coilin layer. The lesions most frequent in the gizzard are the ventriculitis or gizzard inflammation. The most common is the ulcerative ventriculitis, characterised by the presence of ulcers in the gizzard mucosa which may be focalised (fig. 52) or generalised (fig. 53). The presence of ulcers in the gizzard may be associated with starvation conditions, dietary factors, mycotoxins or fungal infections.

## Intestine

The evaluation of the intestine should include the external appearance of the intestinal serosa, the coloration and appearance of the mucosa and the intestinal content. The principal intestinal alterations are:

- Intestinal invagination: it consists of the penetration of one intestinal segment into the lumen of another resulting in necrosis of the intestinal wall. The principal cause is strong intestinal peristalsis often associated with diarrhoea.
- Intestinal obstruction: the partial or total obstruction of the intestinal lumen. This may be due to the impaction of the intestinal contents, an intussusception and, although not common in intensive production poultry, in backyard or extensive breeding flocks it may also be due to a massive parasite infestation, usually nematodes (figs. 54a and 54b).
- Inflammation of the intestine: only enteritis, inflammation of the small intestine, and typhlitis, inflammation of the ceca, are identified in birds. They are distinguished according to the type of exudate/inflammatory infiltrate:

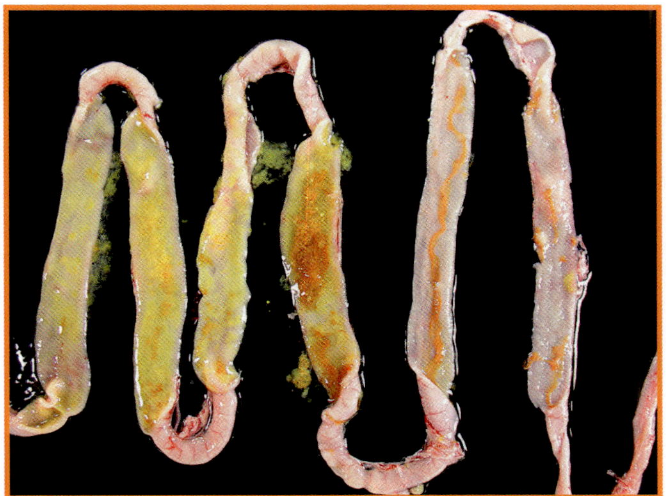

Fig. 55 | Catarrhal enteritis in the jejunum and ileum.

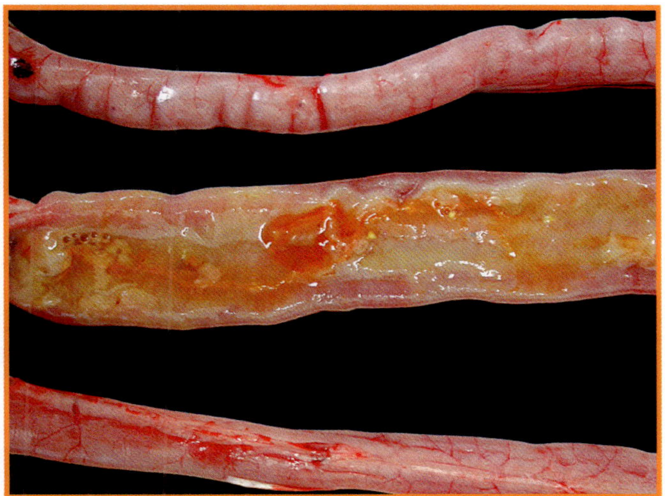

Fig. 56 | Catarrhal enteritis in the jejunum in a case of coccidiosis by *Eimeria maxima*.

- **Catarrhal enteritis.** The term used to describe intestinal disorders in which the intestinal content is more fluid than usual and varied in colour (figs. 55 and 56). Externally, traces of watery diarrhoea in the feathers of the cloaca are seen (fig. 57). It can be caused by an excess secretion (bacterial toxins) or malabsorption and/or poor digestion (nutritional causes, malabsorption syndrome and turkey enteritis). In enteritis caused by *Eimeria acervulina* associated with malabsorption, it is typical to observe white dots in the duodenal mucosa (fig. 58). Occasionally, the presence of nematode parasites can also cause catarrhal enteritis (fig. 59).
- **Ulcerative enteritis.** It is the presence of ulcers in the intestinal mucosa. It is a lesion associated with an infection by *Clostridium colinum* in partridges.
- **Fibrino-necrotic enteritis.** It is characterised by the presence of fibrin in the mucosa and necrosis of the small intestine wall. The most frequent pathology is necrotic enteritis caused by *Clostridium perfringens* (figs. 60 and 61).
- **Hemorrhagic enteritis.** Consists of the presence of blood or bloody content in the small intestine lumen, generally due to necrosis of the wall (figs. 62 and 63). The main cause in birds is coccidiosis by *Eimeria necatrix* (fig. 64), *Eimeria maxima* (figs. 65 and 66), and hemorrhagic turkey enteritis (caused by an adenovirus).
- **Granulomatous enteritis.** It is characterised by the presence of nodules in the intestinal wall. The main causes are bacterial infections, including tuberculosis.

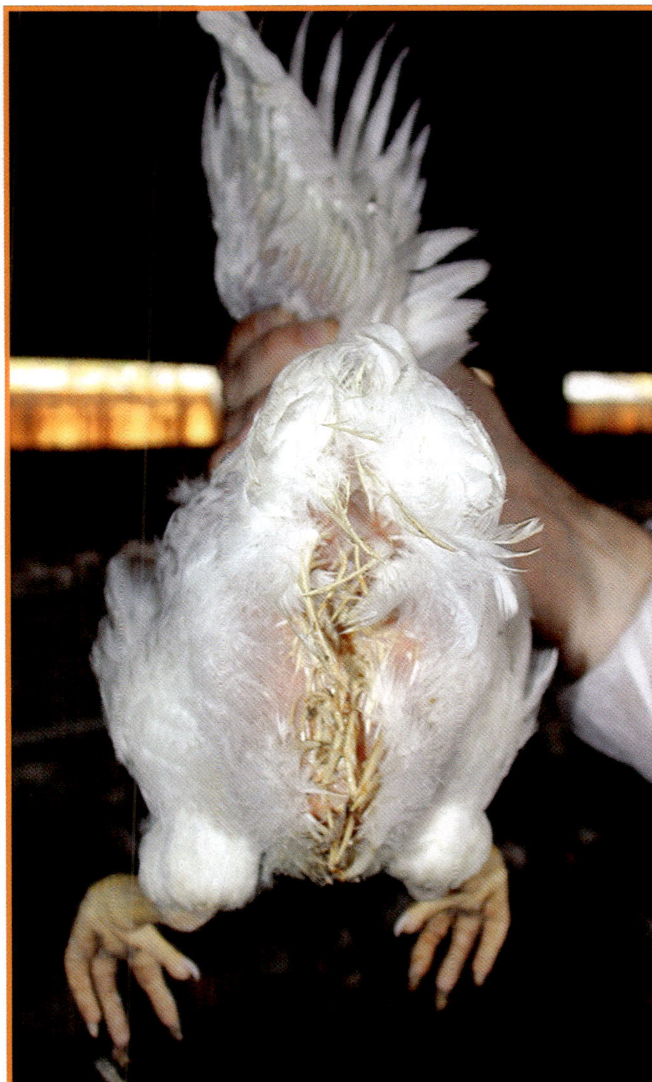

Fig. 57 | Animal with diarrhoea. The presence of faeces on the feathers around the cloaca can be observed.

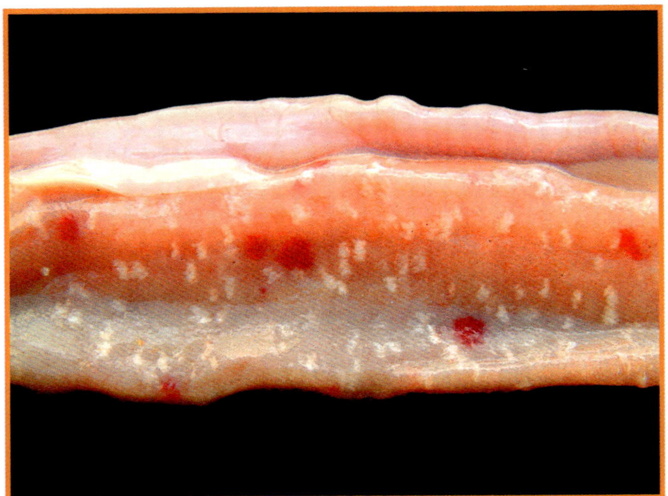
Fig. 58 | Catarrhal enteritis with white dots on the duodenal wall due to infection by *Eimeria acervulina.*

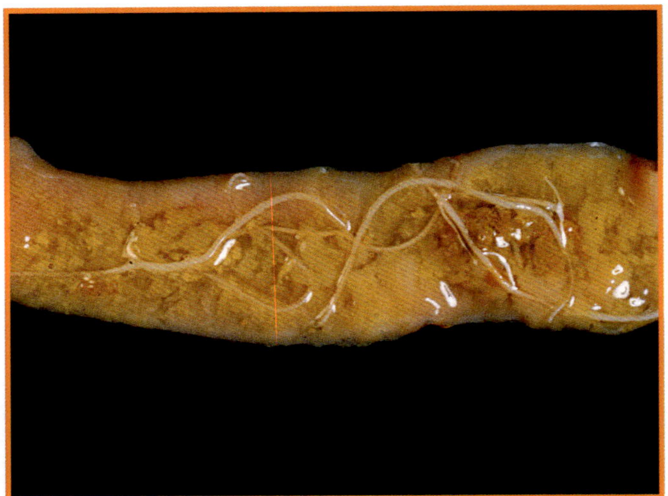
Fig. 59 | Catarrhal enteritis due to parasitic nematodes.

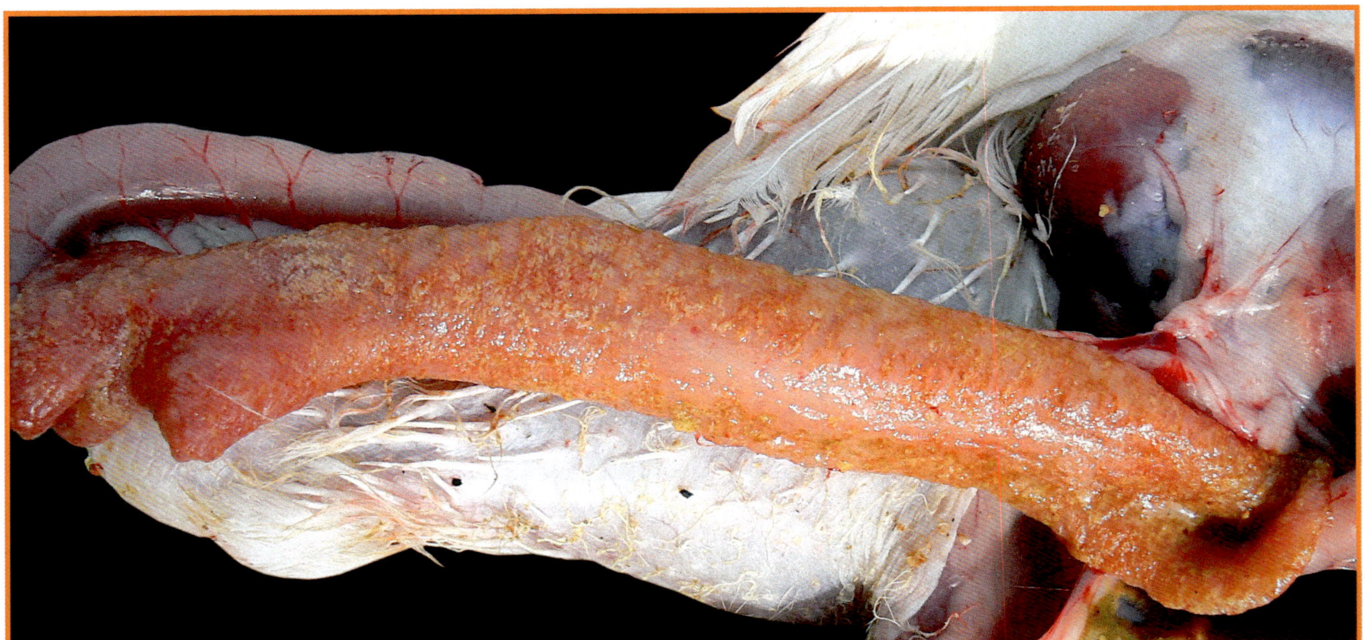
Fig. 60 | Moderate necrotic enteritis where multifocal areas of necrosis in the intestinal mucosa can be observed.

- **Fibrino-necrotic typhlitis.** It is the presence of fibrin on the surface of the mucosa of the ceca. In some cases, fibrin may remain in the lumen and form molds that occupy the intestinal lumen (fig. 67). The main causes of fibrino-necrotic typhlitis are the infections by *Salmonella* spp. and histomoniasis in turkeys.
- **Hemorrhagic typhlitis.** It is characterised by the presence of blood in the intestinal lumen (figs. 68 and 69). Bloody faeces are easily observed in farm surroundings (fig. 70). The main cause is coccidiosis by *Eimeria tenella*.
- **Neoplasia:** the main neoplasia observed in the intestine is lymphoma, caused by Marek's disease virus or avian leukosis.

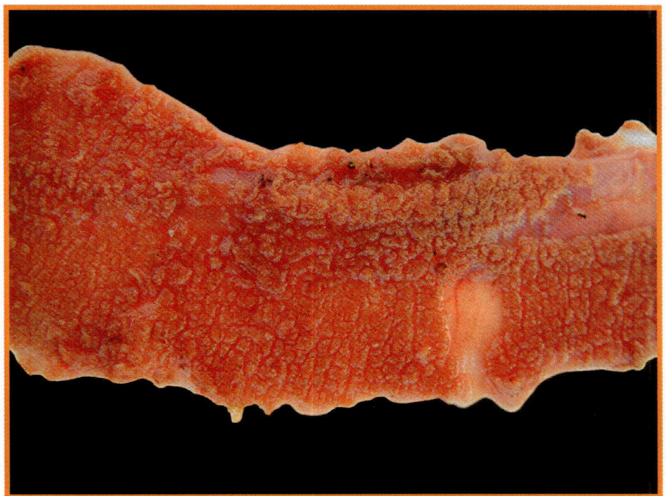

Fig. 61 | Severe necrotic enteritis showing a generalised necrosis of the intestinal mucosa.

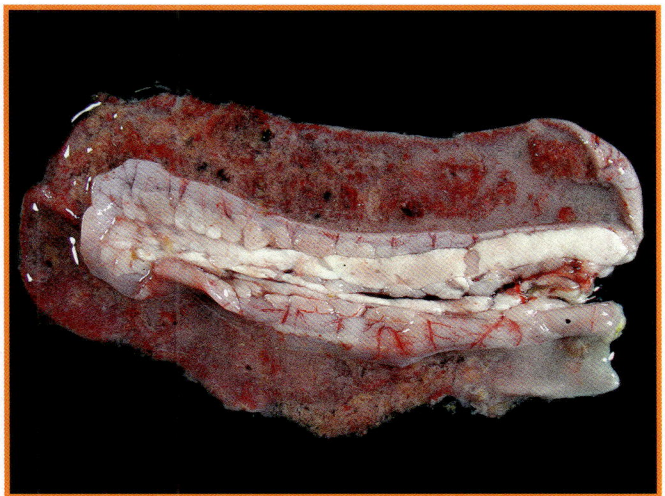

Fig. 62 | Hemorrhagic enteritis in the duodenum.

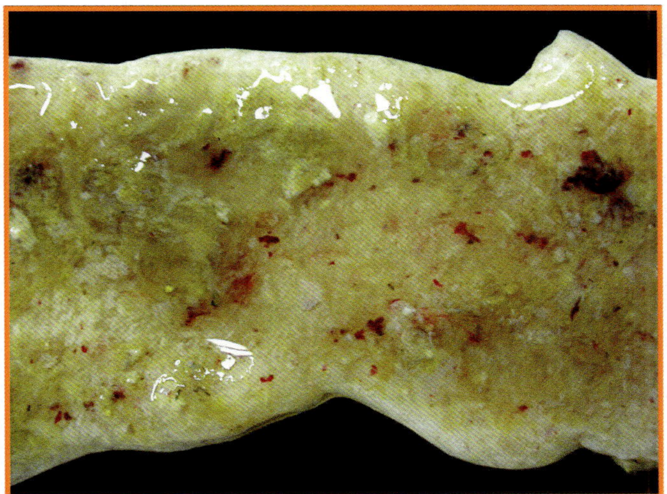

Fig. 63 | Haemorrhagic enteritis in the jejunum of a breeder chick due to coccidiosis.

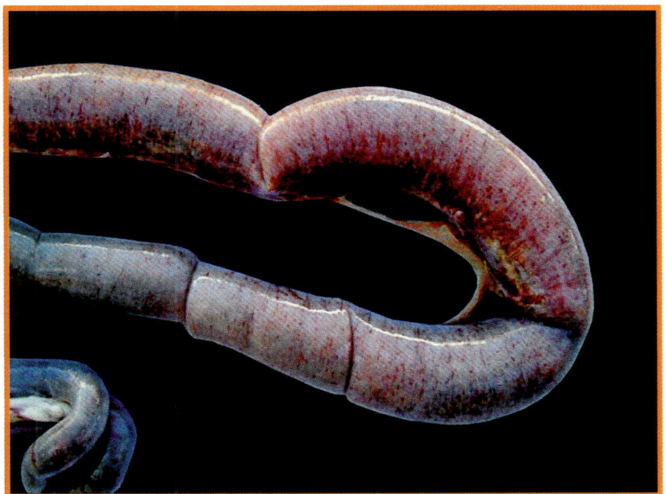

Fig. 64 | Hemorrhagic enteritis in the jejunum due to coccidiosis by *Eimeria necatrix*.

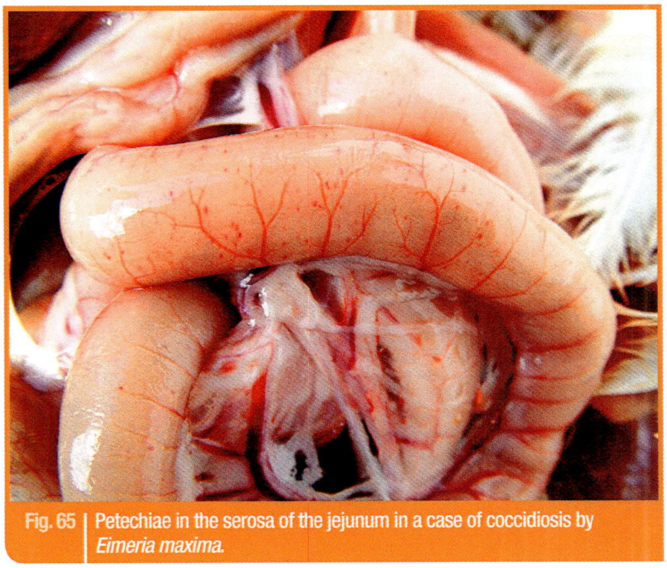

Fig. 65 | Petechiae in the serosa of the jejunum in a case of coccidiosis by *Eimeria maxima*.

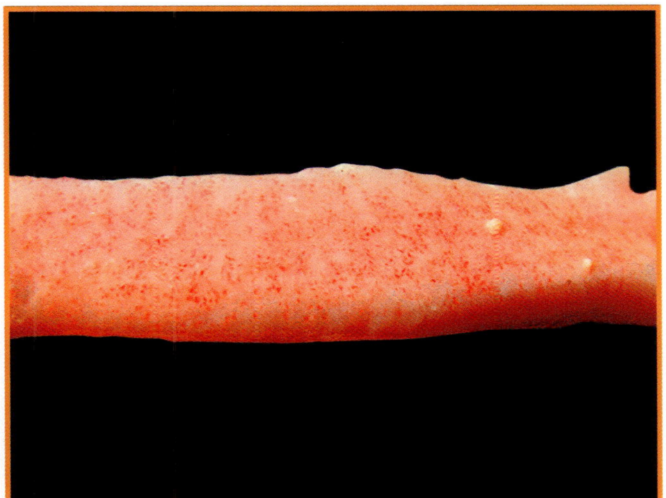

Fig. 66 | Moderate hemorrhagic enteritis with petechiae generalised throughout the mucosa of the jejunum, in a case of coccidiosis by *Eimeria maxima*.

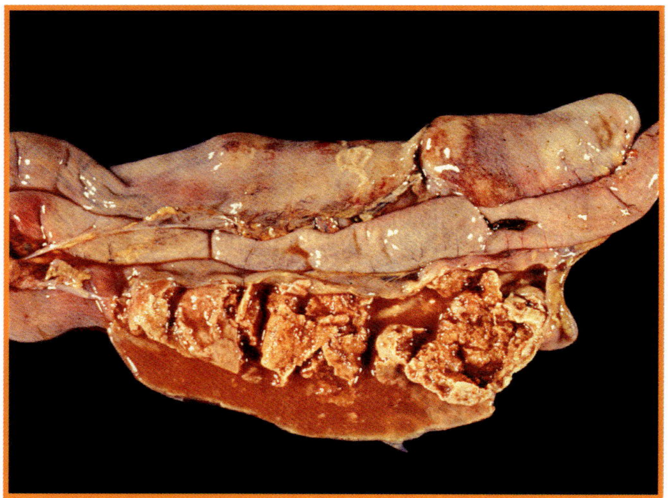
Fig. 67 | Fibrino-necrotic typhlitis presenting caseous material in the ceca lumen in a case of histomoniasis.

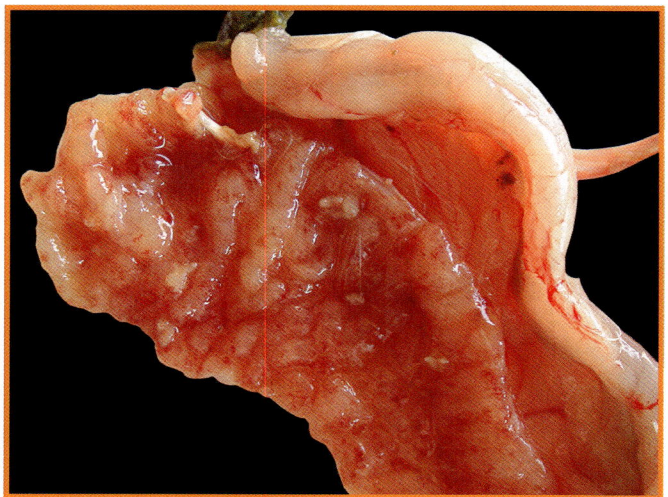
Fig. 68 | Moderate haemorrhagic typhlitis in a case of coccidiosis by *Eimeria tenella.*

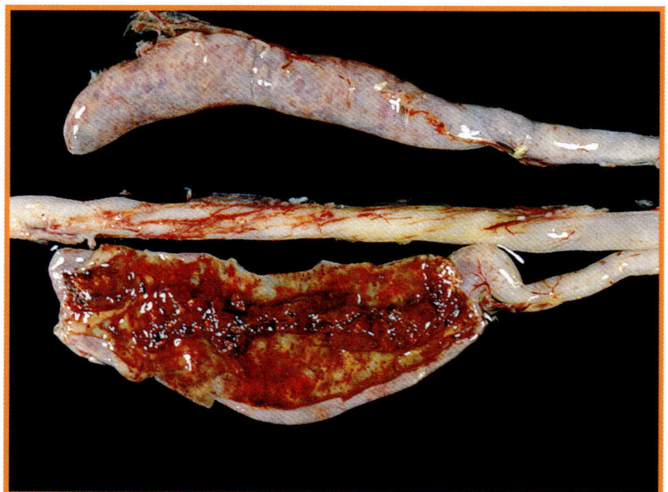
Fig. 69 | Severe haemorrhagic typhlitis in a case of coccidiosis by *Eimeria tenella.*

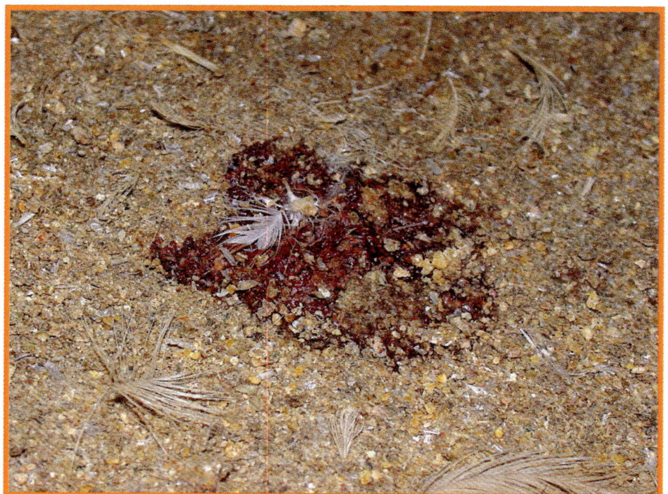
Fig. 70 | Bloody droppings in a batch affected by coccidiosis caused by *Eimeria tenella.*

## Pancreas

The pancreas is an organ in which virtually no gross lesions are evident. In some cases it is possible to observe generalised whitish dots in the pancreatic parenchyma which usually has no pathological significance. The primary lesion is pancreatic necrosis (fig. 71) characterised by the presence of haemorrhages in the pancreatic parenchyma and mainly associated with an avian influenza or Newcastle virus infection.

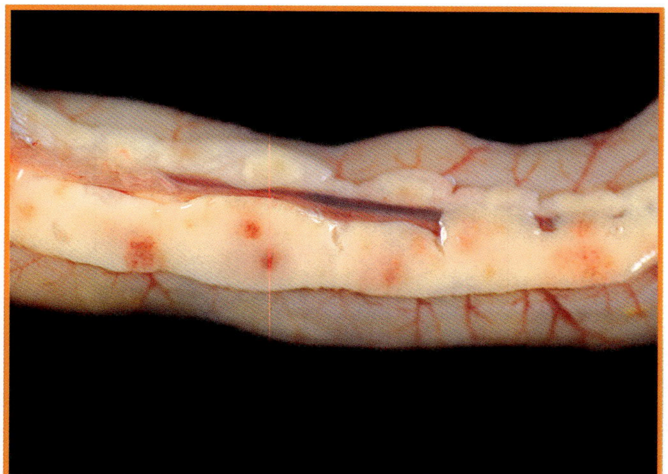
Fig. 71 | Pancreatic necrosis characterised by haemorrhages in the pancreatic parenchyma in an animal infected by a highly pathogenic avian influenza virus.

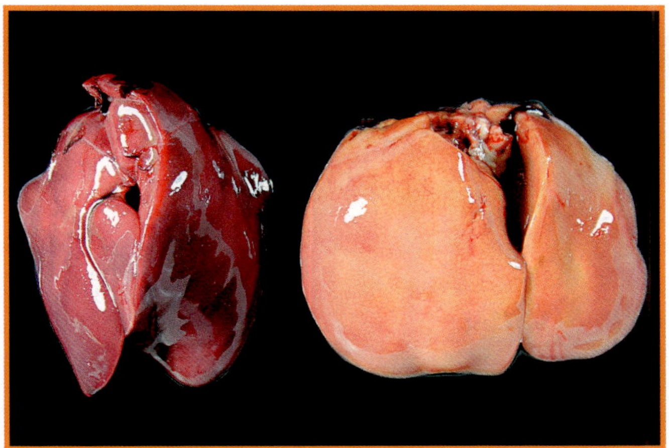

Fig. 72 | Hepatic lipidosis. The liver on the right shows hepatic lipidosis. The increase in size and pale discoloration is considerable when compared to a normal liver (left).

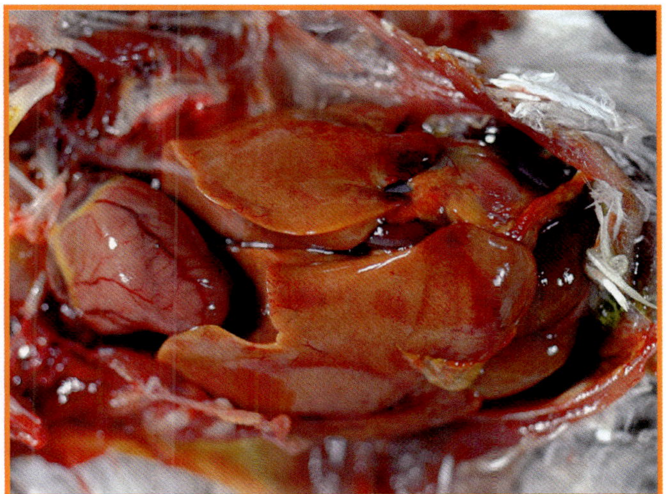

Fig. 73 | Hepatic amyloidosis.

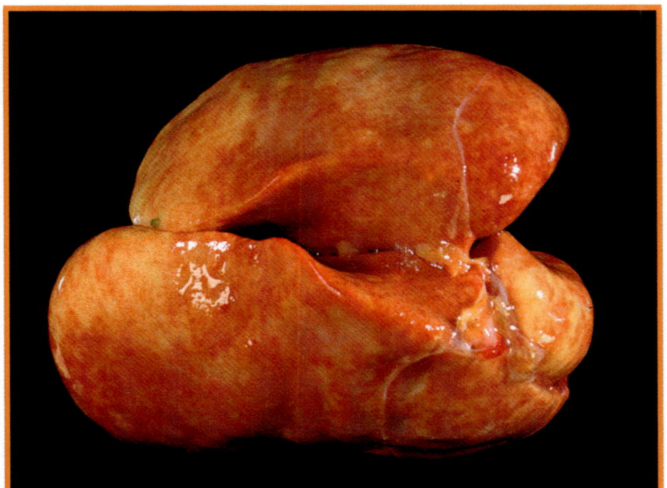

Fig. 74 | Hepatic fibrosis and lipidosis in a bird affected by ascites. The liver is decreased in size, its capsule is thicker and it is notably pale.

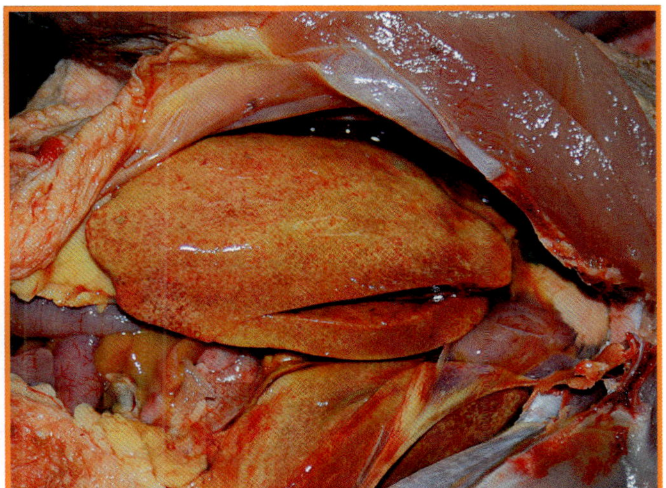

Fig. 75 | Petechial haemorrage and significant hepatic pallor in a bird affected by inclusion body hepatitis.

## Liver

The liver is the largest organ of the coelomic cavity and, consequently, the person performing the necropsy usually examines it carefully. It should be highlighted that, in general, there are few pathological processes that cause specific macroscopic lesions in the liver and a microscopic examination is necessary to be able to determine the nature of the lesion.

The macroscopic evaluation of the liver should include **the size**, **the coloration** and **the consistency**. The major pathological processes that affect the liver include:

- **Lipidosis and steatosis:** it is a lipid accumulation in the cytoplasm of the hepatocytes which causes a diffuse yellow coloration, an increase in size and a decreased consistency of the liver (fig. 72). This lesion is associated with fatty liver and kidney syndrome in chickens, fatty liver haemorrhagic syndrome in laying hens or to mycotoxicosis. It may also be observed in conditions of high energetic/metabolic demand or the event of starvation.
- **Amyloidosis:** it is the deposition of amyloid material (protein) in the hepatic parenchyma. Macroscopically, the liver has a similar appearance to a liver with hepatic lipidosis: an increase in size and yellowing but with normal consistency (fig. 73). It is often observed in animals affected by chronic systemic infections (colibacillosis, tuberculosis, etc.).

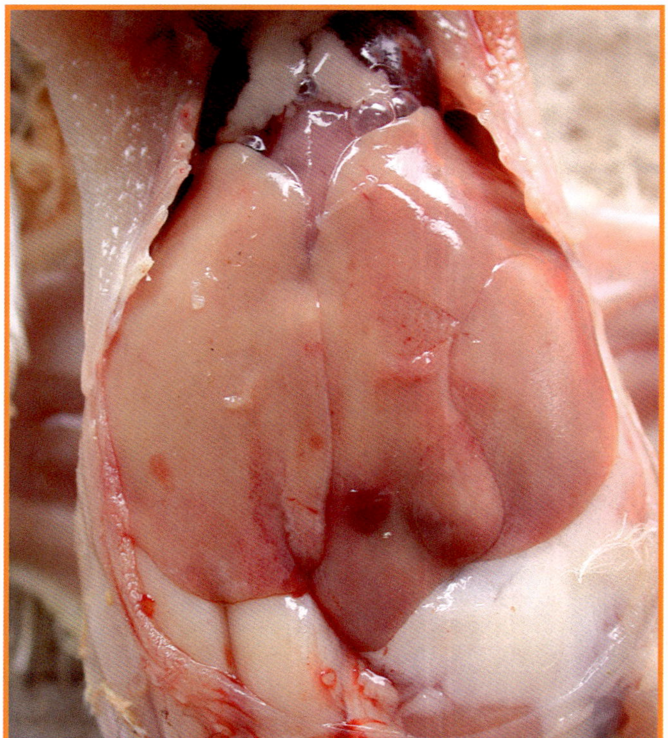

Fig. 76 | Small subcapsular haematoma in a bird with hepatic lipidosis.

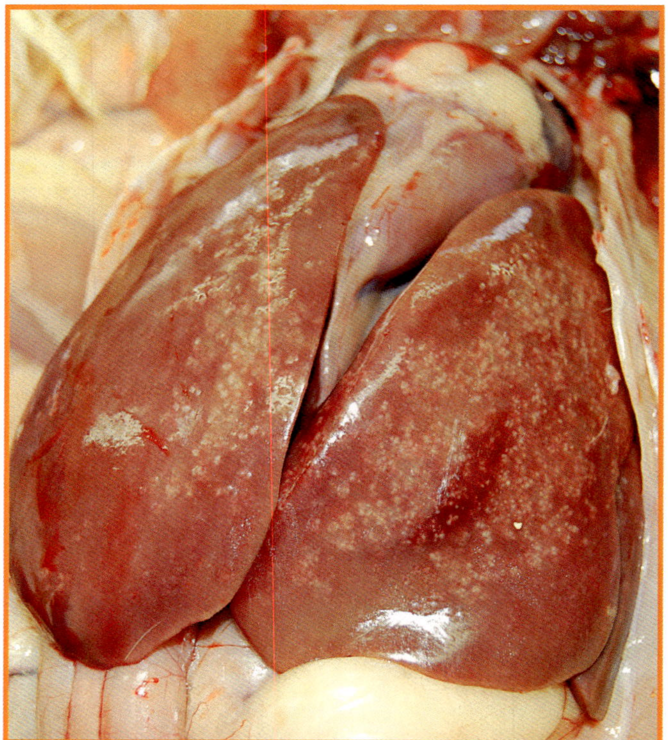

Fig. 77 | Multifocal necrotising hepatitis associated with bacterial septicaemia.

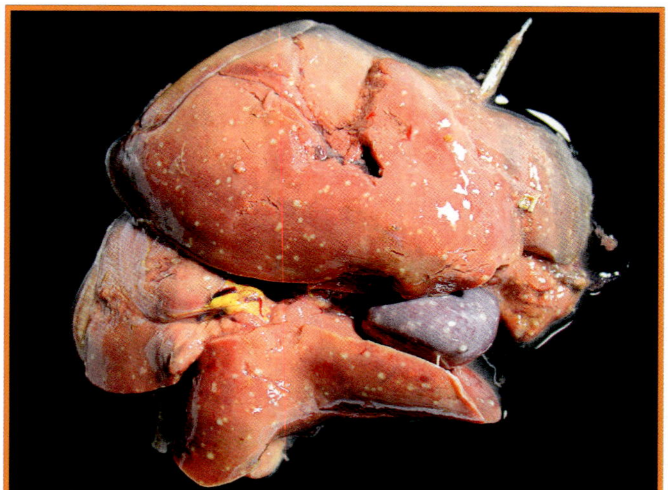

Fig. 78 | Multifocal necrotising hepatitis associated with bacterial septicaemia.

- **Fibrosis:** this lesion causes a decrease in liver size, which appears contracted, including an increased consistency and a marked thickening of the capsule (fig. 74). It is a very nonspecific lesion because it can be associated with different diagnoses such as ascites or chronic poisoning.
- **Haemorrhages:** this is a lesion that is observed relatively frequently. It can occur as multiple petechiae or ecchymosis affecting the surface, but also affecting the hepatic parenchyma (fig. 75). This type of lesion is usually caused by viral infections (inclusion body hepatitis in chickens or haemorrhagic turkey enteritis) or mycotoxicoses. Other forms of presentation are subcapsular haemorrhages or haematomas (fig. 76) which may be more or less extensive and are associated with trauma. The decrease in hepatic consistency due to hepatic lipidosis, for example, may promote the appearance of this lesion.
- **Perihepatitis:** it is the presence of fibrinous exudate on the surface of the liver. It is usually seen in cases of fibrinous polyserositis caused by bacterial sepsis.
- **Hepatitis:** the hepatic inflammation, usually associated with necrosis, presents different gross images. On occasion, especially in cases of inclusion body hepatitis, the hepatic parenchyma is pale in colour and, as already mentioned, petechiae or haemorrages are seen (fig. 75). In cases of hepatitis caused by bacterial sepsis, multiple whitish foci of necrosis distributed throughout the hepatic parenchyma are frequently observed (figs. 77 and 78). In the case of turkeys, histomoniasis produces hepatitis le-

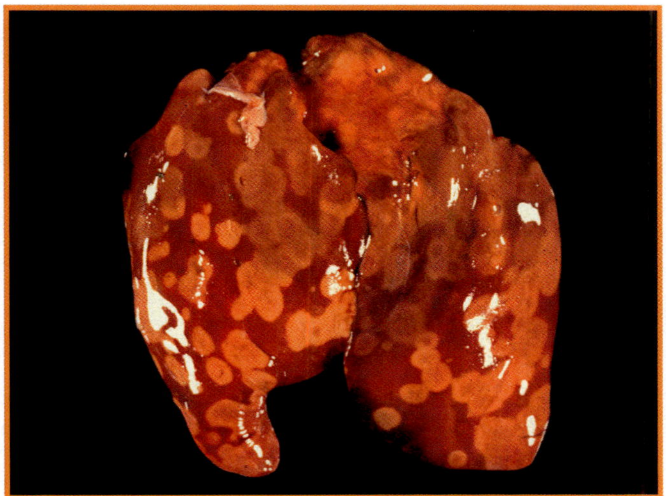

Fig. 79 | Necrotising hepatitis associated with *Histomonas meleagridis* in turkeys.

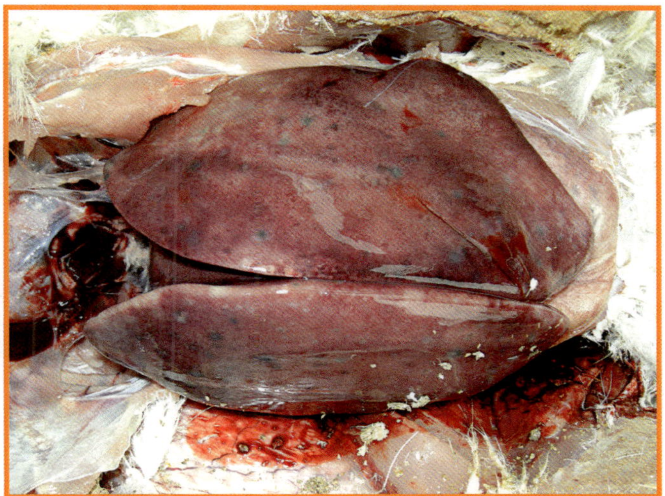

Fig. 80 | Hepatic lymphoma in a case of lymphoproliferative disease in turkeys.

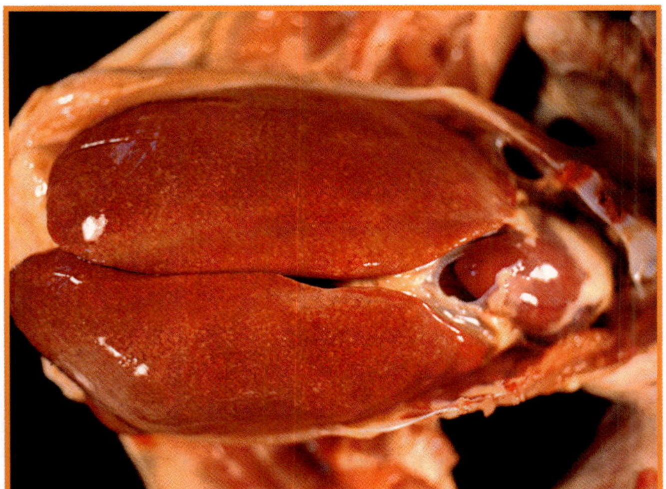

Fig. 81 | Hepatic lymphoma showing the significant enlargement of the liver and generalised white dots in a case of avian leukosis.

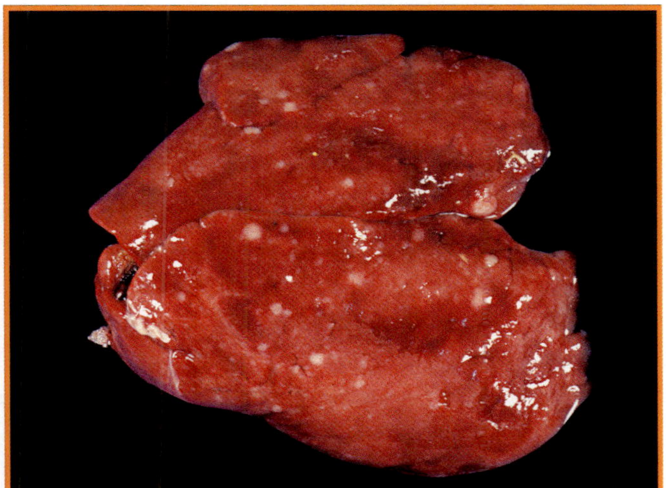

Fig. 82 | Hepatic lymphoma in the form of multiple white nodules, caused by Marek's disease virus.

sions with yellowish foci and a darker central area (fig. 79). A particular type of hepatic inflammation is cholangiohepatitis, usually caused by *Clostridium perfringens*. This gross lesion of the liver varies, but often a thickening of the gallbladder wall is observed.

- **Neoplasia:** lymphoma is the neoplasia which most frequently affects the liver and is associated with Marek's disease as well as avian leukosis or lymphoproliferative disease in turkeys (fig. 80). These diseases can cause lymphomas, presented as white, multifocal areas of varying size (figs. 81 and 82) or as a diffuse increase in the size of the liver (fig. 83).

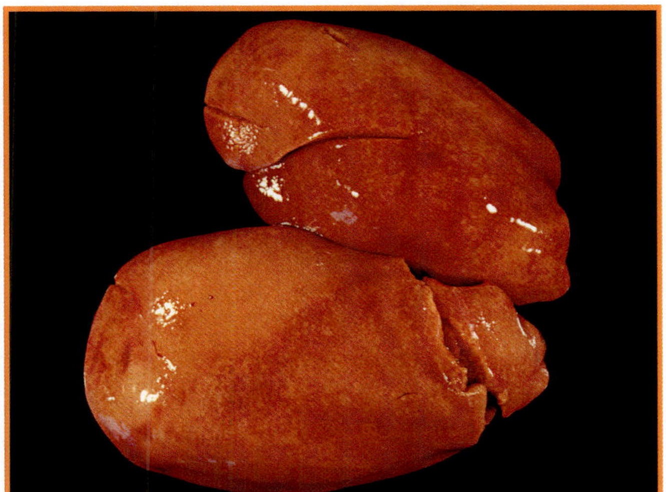

Fig. 83 | Hepatic lymphoma with a notably enlarged liver in a case of avian leukosis.

# Cardiovascular system

This section includes lesions which affect the heart and larger vessels. The heart of a bird, unlike mammals, is conical-shaped with a left/right ventricle thickness proportion of 1:4 (the left being the largest). As discussed in Chapter 1, the examination of the heart is achieved by performing a cross section at ventricle level.

Some of the major pathological disorders which affect the cardiovascular system are:

- **Pulmonary hypertension syndrome:** the principal associated lesion is ascites (fig. 84), as a consequence of right-sided heart failure, secondary to pulmonary hypertension. This syndrome is associated with rapid growth, fattening conditions at higher altitudes or even sodium poisoning. Ascitis is characterised by an accumulation of serous fluid in the coelomic cavity. In addition, a significant dilatation and hypertrophy of the right ventricular wall can be observed (fig. 85) in response to pulmonary hypertension and in some cases, hydropericardium.

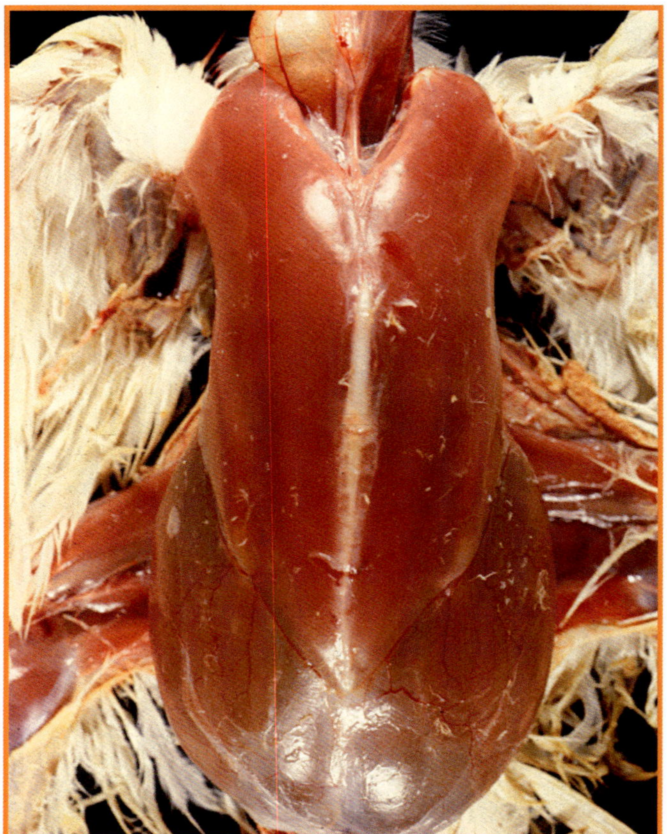

Fig. 84 | Animal with ascites characterised by abundant serous fluid in the coelomic cavity.

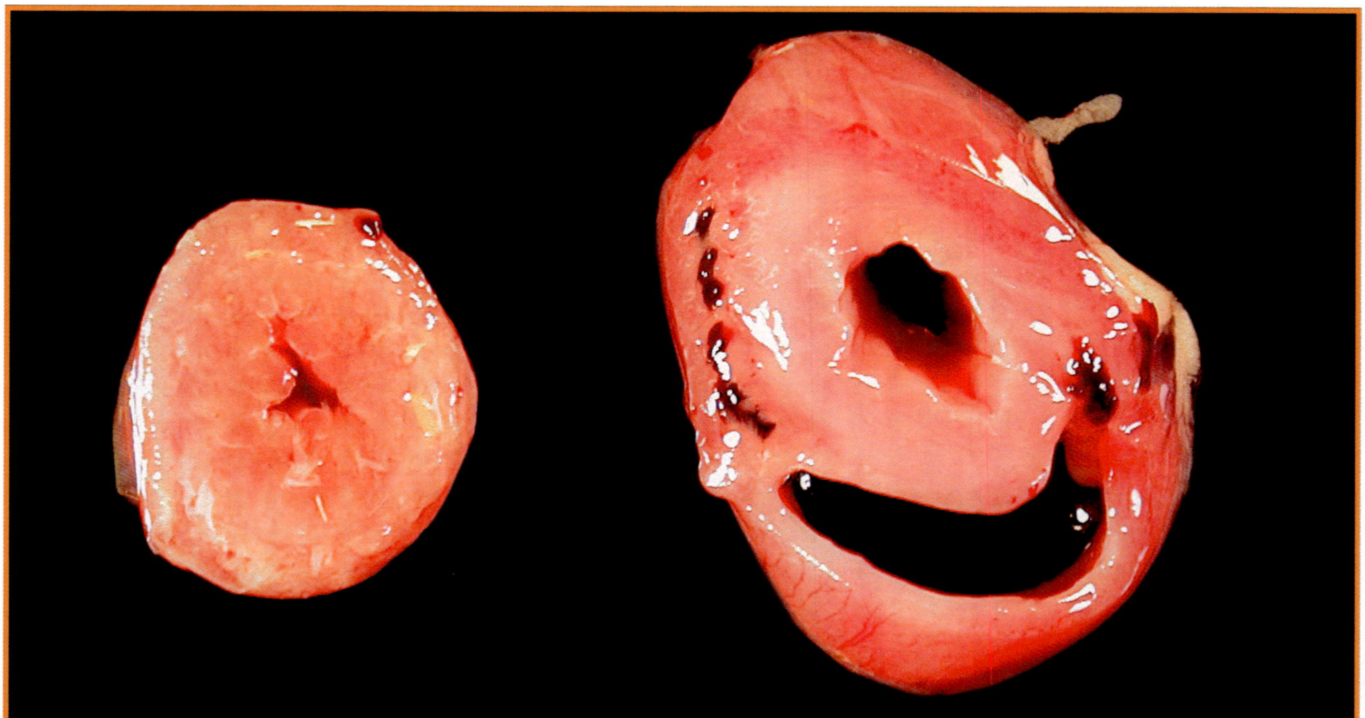

Fig. 85 | Cross sections of the heart. The right section corresponds to an animal with significant dilation and hypertrophy of the right ventricle. The left section corresponds to a healthy animal.

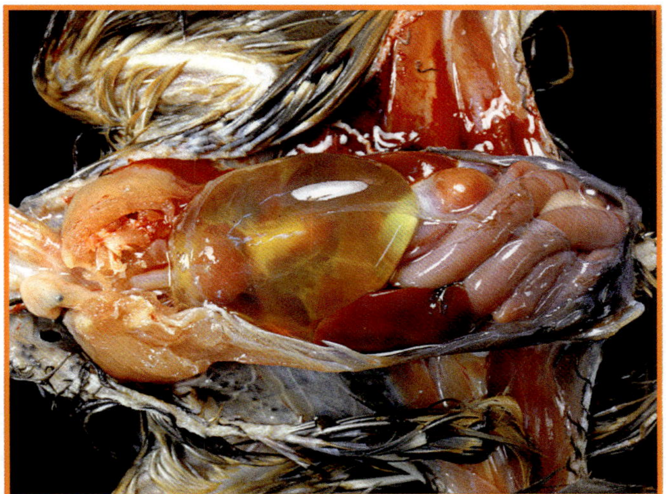

Fig. 86 | Hydropericardium.

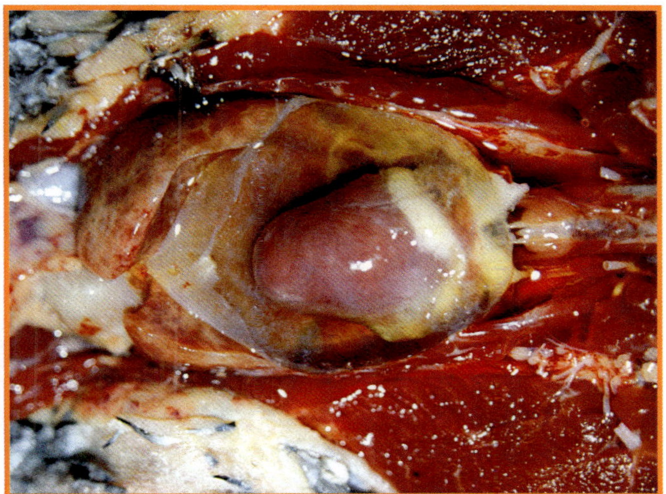

Fig. 87 | Hydropericardium.

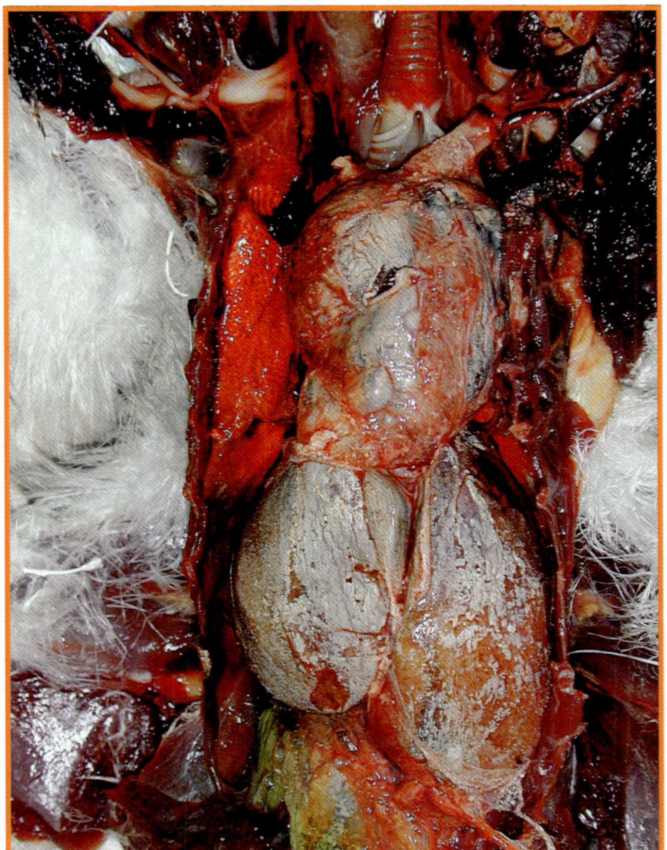

Fig. 88 | Visceral gout is characterised by a whitish deposition (urate crystals) in the serous membranes of the coelomic cavity.

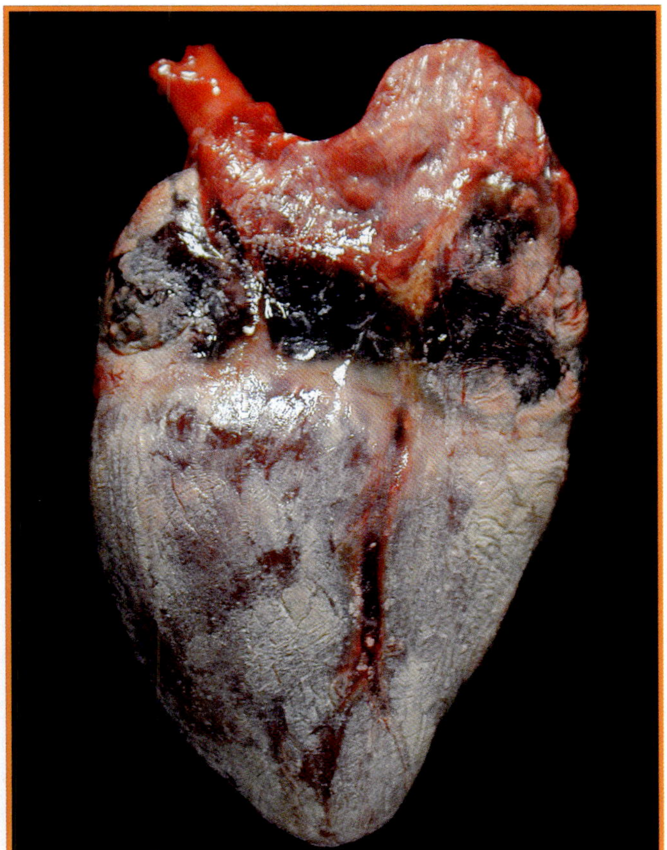

Fig. 89 | Visceral gout affecting the pericardium.

- **Hydropericardium:** this lesion is the accumulation of serous fluid in the pericardial cavity (figs. 86 and 87). In most cases it is associated with ascites and heart failure, but it is also seen in inclusion body hepatitis caused by an adenovirus.
- **Visceral gout:** it is produced by the deposition of uric acid crystals identified as white granular material in the pericardium. It is generally associated with impaired renal function (figs. 88 and 89).

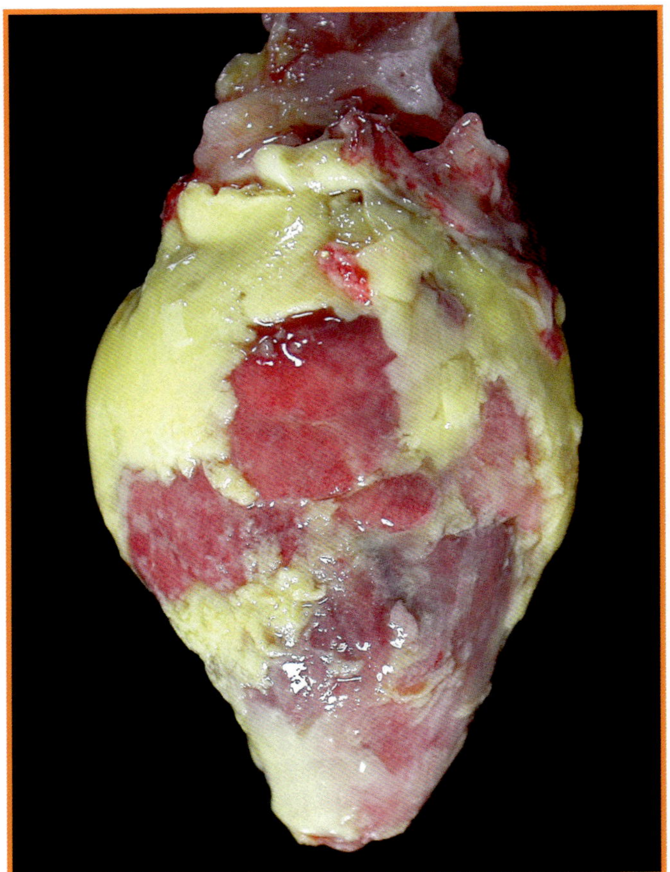

Fig. 90 | Fibrinous pericarditis showing the presence of fibrinous exudate on the pericardial surface.

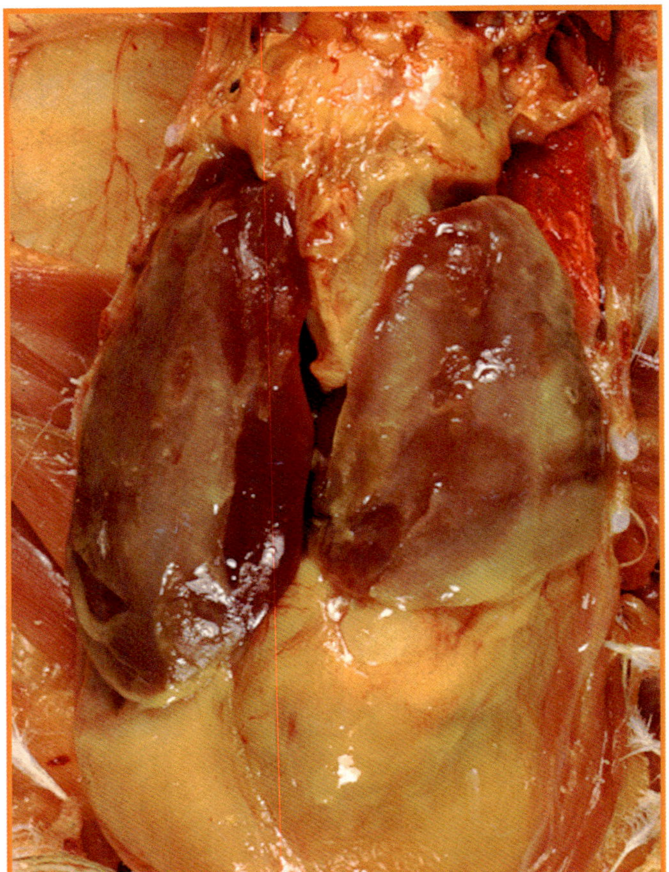

Fig. 91 | Fibrinous polyserositis with fibrin exudate on the serous membranes of the coelomic cavity.

- **Pericarditis:** it is an inflammation of the serous membranes surrounding the heart and forming the pericardium sac. This lesion is characterised by the presence of exudate, usually fibrinous or fibrinopurulent, in the pericardial cavity or on the surface of the visceral pericardium (fig. 90). This lesion is frequent in animals suffering from septicaemia, usually due to *Escherichia coli*. It is normal to observe perihepatitis and airsacculitis (polyserositis) in addition to pericarditis (fig. 91).
- **Neoplasm of the myocardium:** it is relatively rare, but the most common tumour is lymphoma, seen as white areas or nodules in the myocardium (fig. 92) associated to Marek's disease virus.
- **Aortic rupture in turkeys:** it is an uncommon lesion but can lead to elevated mortality losses in male turkeys. The rupture of the aorta and subsequent massive haemorrhage in the coelomic cavity often originates from an aneurysm which forms in the abdominal aorta and produces the bird's death.

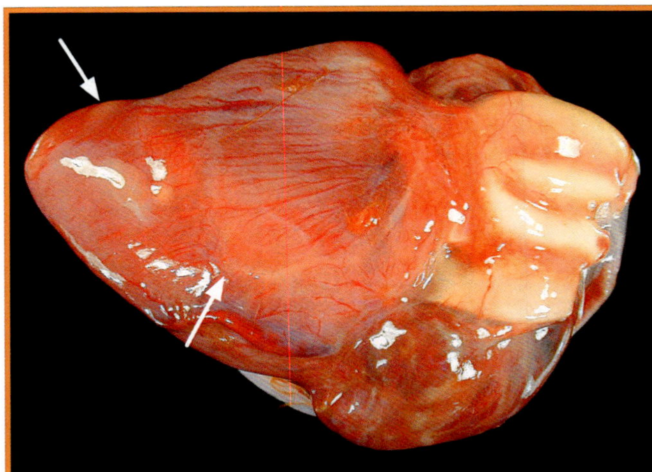

Fig. 92 | Myocardial lymphoma in a bird affected by an acute or visceral form (arrows) of Marek's disease.

# Lymphohaematopoietic system

Included in this section are the lesions affecting the thymus, spleen and bursa of Fabricius. The most important characteristics to be assessed in these organs are the size and coloration. It is important to note that, as discussed above, both the thymus and the bursa of Fabricius are organs that regress with age. Therefore the size, which is one of the most important parameters to grossly evaluate these organs, varies considerably depending on the age of the bird.

## Thymus

The principal gross lesion in this organ is a notable decrease in size known as thymic atrophy (fig. 93). This is a significant lesion in broilers and may have multiple causes, but the most common cause is an infection by avian infectious anaemia virus. Usually this disease causes pale pink or yellowish lesions in the affected animal's bone marrow (fig. 94). Haemorrhaging, normally observed due to the presence of petechiae, is often found in the thymus although it is nonspecific.

## Spleen

Like the thymus, a change in size is the most common gross alteration to be observed. An increase in the relative size of the spleen, known as splenomegaly, is normal as a primary response to circulating antigen. This size increase is usually accompanied by miliary white spots seen both on the organ surface as well as at the section (fig. 95). This lesion is often observed in animals suffering from septicaemia, mainly due to *Escherichia coli*.

Inflammation of the spleen, known as splenitis, is quite rare. It is seen in cases of tuberculosis in which the spleen has multiple white nodules that correspond to granulomas (fig. 96).

Finally, the spleen may be enlarged due to the presence of a lymphoma in animals affected by Marek's disease or avian leukosis (fig. 97).

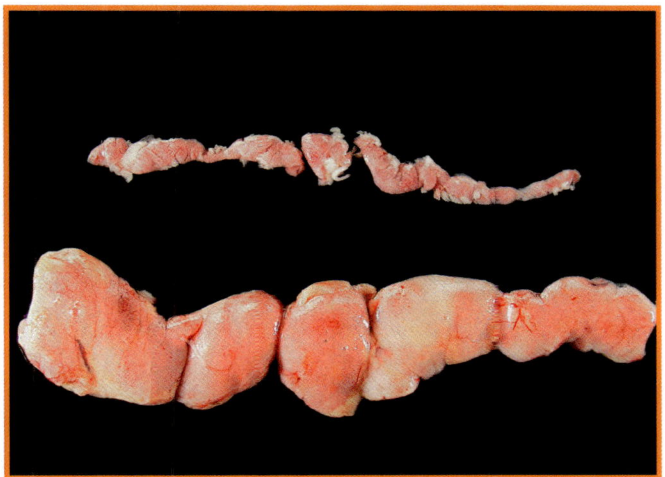

Fig. 93 | Marked thymic atrophy in a bird affected by avian infectious anaemia.

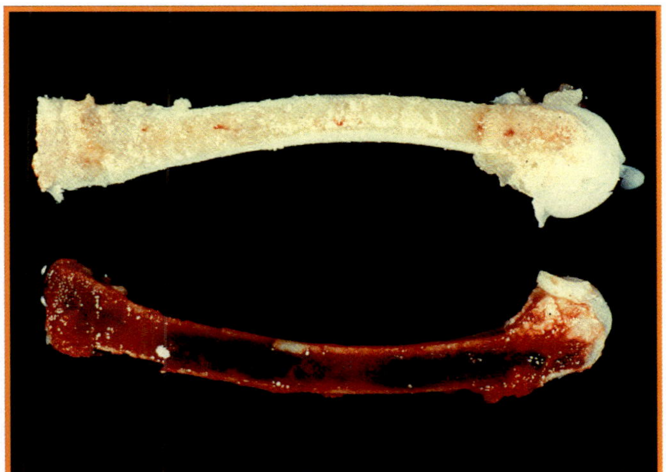

Fig. 94 | The femur bone marrow is significantly pale in a bird affected by avian infectious anaemia.

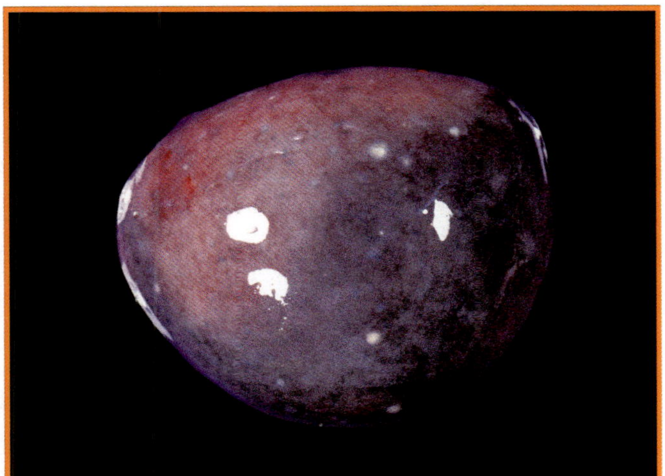

Fig. 95 | Splenomegaly in a bird affected by colisepticaemia.

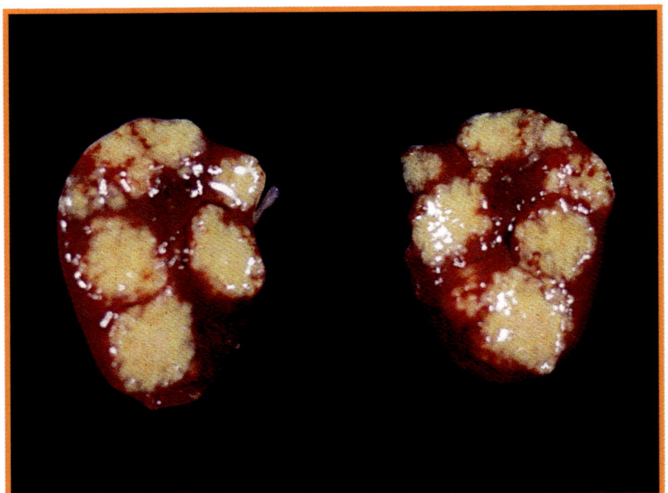

Fig. 96 | Granulomatous splenitis in a bird with avian tuberculosis.

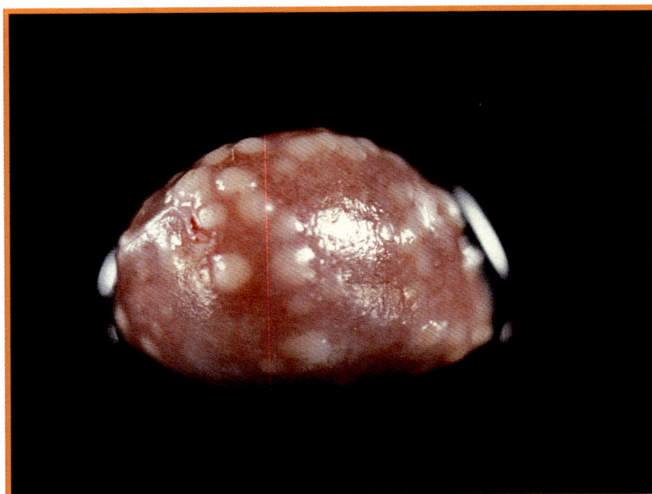

Fig. 97 | A splenic lymphoma with multiple white nodules in a bird affected by avian leukosis.

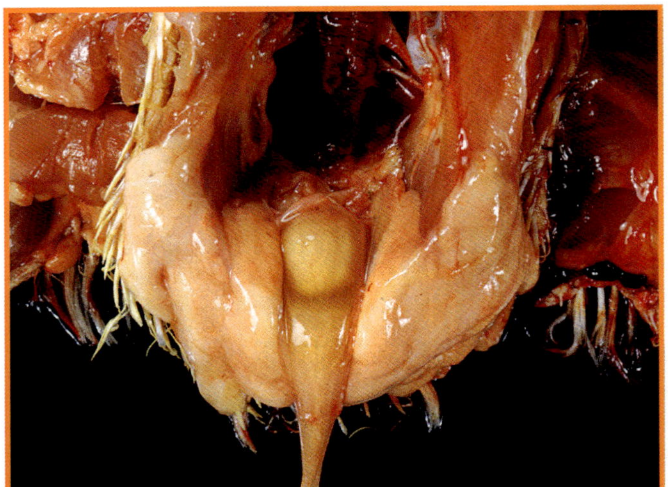

Fig. 98 | A significant enlargement of the bursa of Fabricius as well as a peribursal oedema in a bird affected by IBD (Gumboro disease).

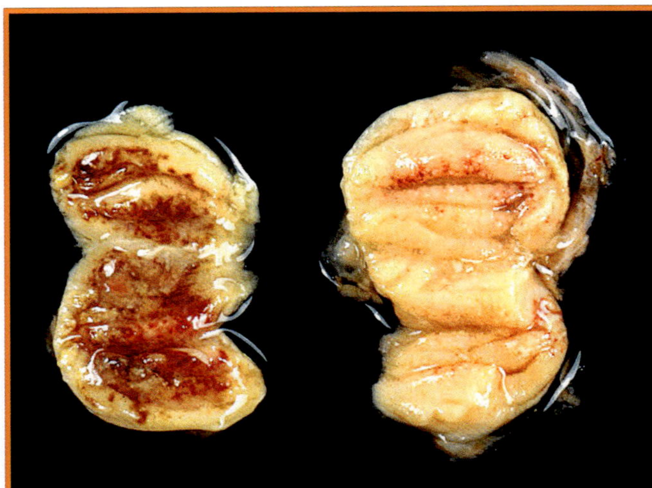

Fig. 99 | Diffuse petechial haemorrhages, in the bursae of Fabricius of birds affected by IBD (Gumboro disease).

## Bursa of Fabricius

As in the two organs mentioned above, a change in the size of the bursa is one of the most important lesions to evaluate together with changes in coloration.

The decrease in size of the bursa or atrophy is a fairly non-specific lesion. It may be caused by nutritional deficiencies, mycotoxin ingestion or even viral infections such as Marek's disease or avian reovirosis. Occasionally a significant atrophy of the bursa of Fabricius may be observed in animals infected with IBD (Gumboro disease) virus.

As for an increase in the size of the bursa, this may be due either to an inflammation, known as bursitis, or to the presence of a neoplasm, usually lymphoma. Bursitis is observed mainly in animals suffering from acute IBD (Gumboro disease), and the enlargement of the bursa is associated with inflammatory changes, such as peribursal and intrabursal oedemas (fig. 98), and haemorrhage, appearing as petechiae or diffusely affecting the whole bursa (fig. 99). Sporadically, bursa oedema and haemorrhage may be caused by bacteria, and this should not be confused with IBD (Gumboro disease). The bursa of Fabricius affected by lymphoma normally shows a greater enlargement than in bursitis and suffers no change of colour. The most common cause of bursa lymphoma is avian leukosis, which may also affect the spleen, liver and other organs.

# Genitourinary system

This section includes the lesions that affect the urinary system and the reproductive system.

## Urinary System

The urinary system consists of the kidneys and ureters which empty into the cloaca. As discussed in Chapter 1, the kidneys should be evaluated in situ in the coelomic cavity. This evaluation should take into account the **size and colour** of the kidneys, **depositions** on the renal surface or parenchyma, as well as **urate retention**.

It should be remembered that in some cases, the increased renal size and pallor may not be associated with histological lesions. For example, autolysis of the kidneys may lead to colour changes which can be misleading (fig. 100).

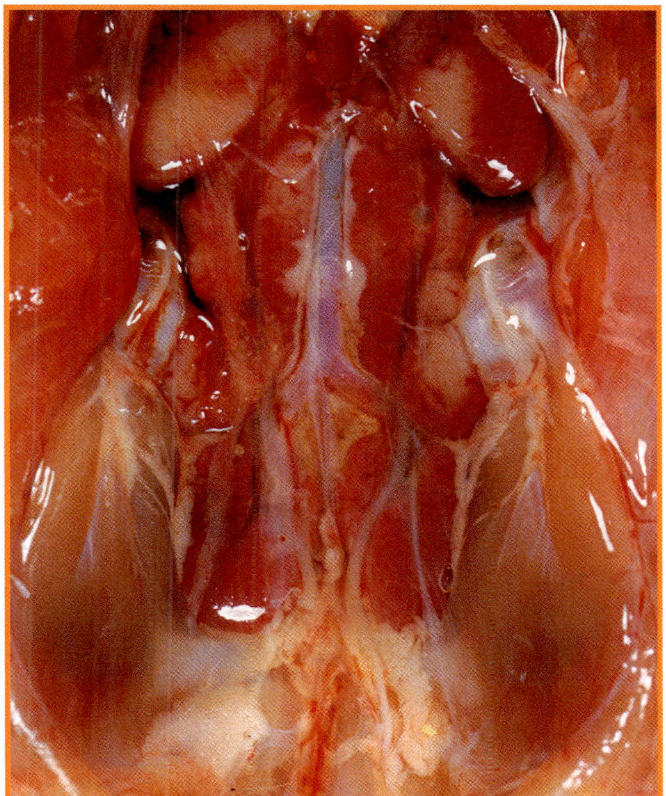

Fig. 100 | Multiple areas of renal pallor in a bird in an advanced state of autolysis.

In general, there are not many changes observable in the kidneys and different pathologies coincide in the same gross image. The main renal alterations are summarised as follows:

- **Renal agenesis:** it is a congenital malformation characterised by the absence of one of the two kidneys (fig. 101). It is generally considered a necropsy finding without major clinical consequences.
- **Nephritis:** this is inflammation of the kidney. It may be primary, due to viral infections, which are the most common causes (infectious bronchitis virus, avian influenza virus and Newcastle virus, among other agents), or bacterial infections (erysipelas, *Streptococcus* spp. or *Pasteurella*). Early stages show renal pallor (fig. 102) and nephromegaly, and in later stages urate accumulation in the kidneys may be evident (fig. 103). In cases of renal tubular damage triggered by dehydration (caused by water deprivation or febrile infections), the appearance of the kidneys is practically the same (figs. 104 and 105). A specific type of nephritis is granulomatous nephritis, characterised by the presence of granulomas in the renal parenchyma. Macroscopically the tumours cannot be differentiated, however, histologically fungal forms are seen in the interior of the granulomas. They are mostly respiratory fungal infections which spread to the kidneys by contact through the air sacs (fig. 106).

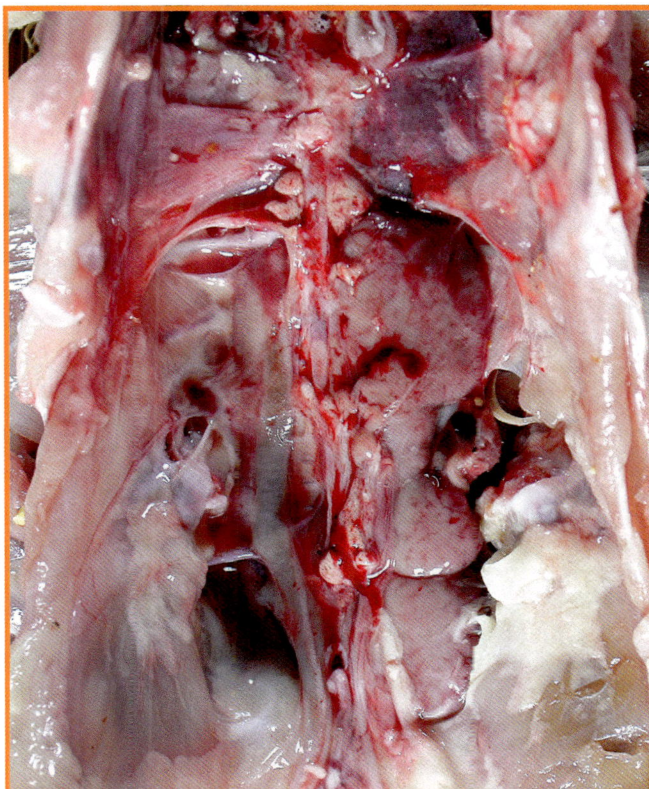

Fig. 101 | Renal agenesis. The absence of the right kidney is shown.

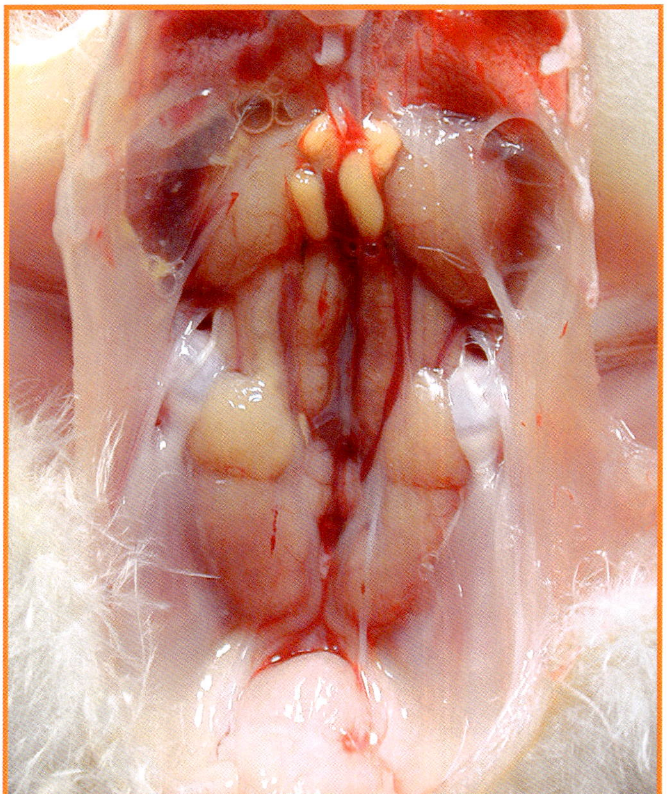

Fig. 102 | Nephritis characterised by renal pallor in a bird infected with avian infectious bronchitis.

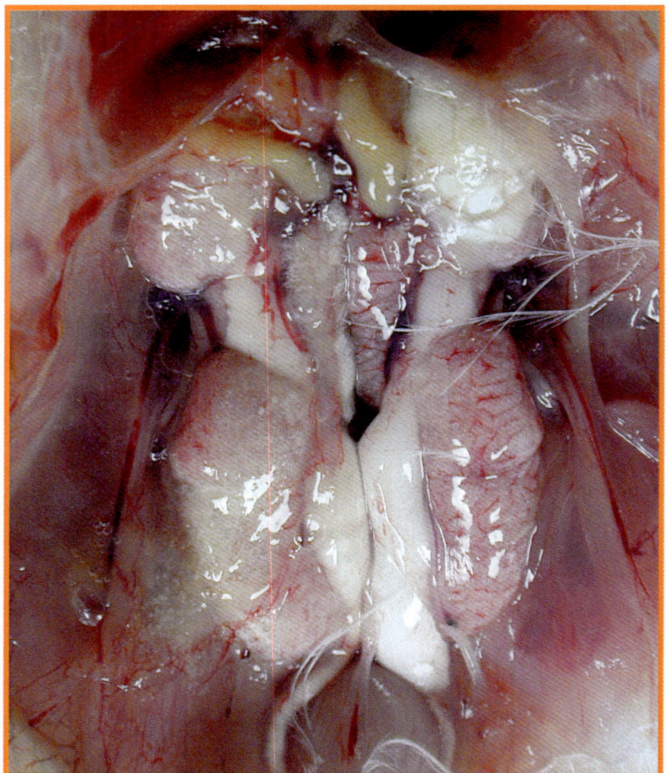

Fig. 103 | Nephritis with enlarged kidneys and an accumulation of urates in the kidneys and ureters, in a bird infected with avian infectious bronchitis.

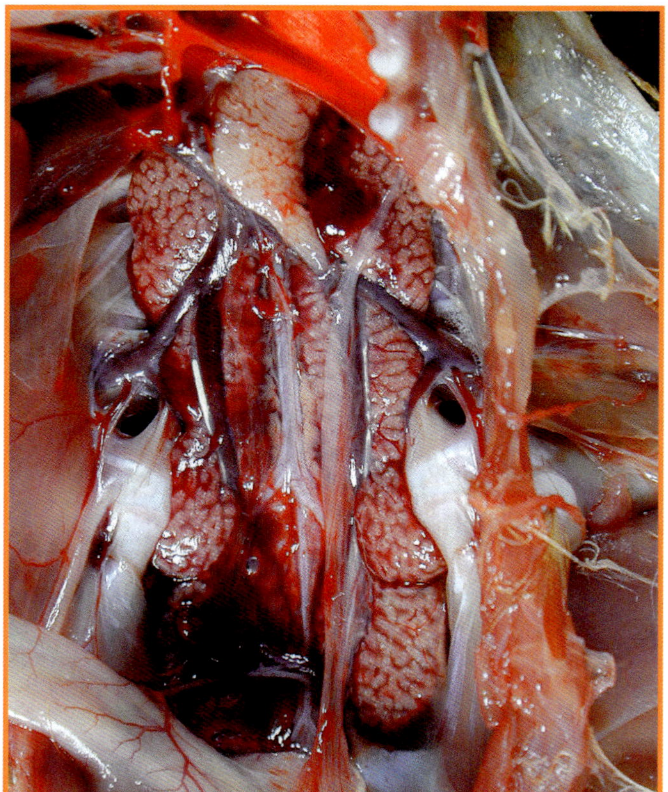

Fig. 104 | Nephritis with renal pallor and an accumulation of urates in the kidneys of a bird suffering dehydration.

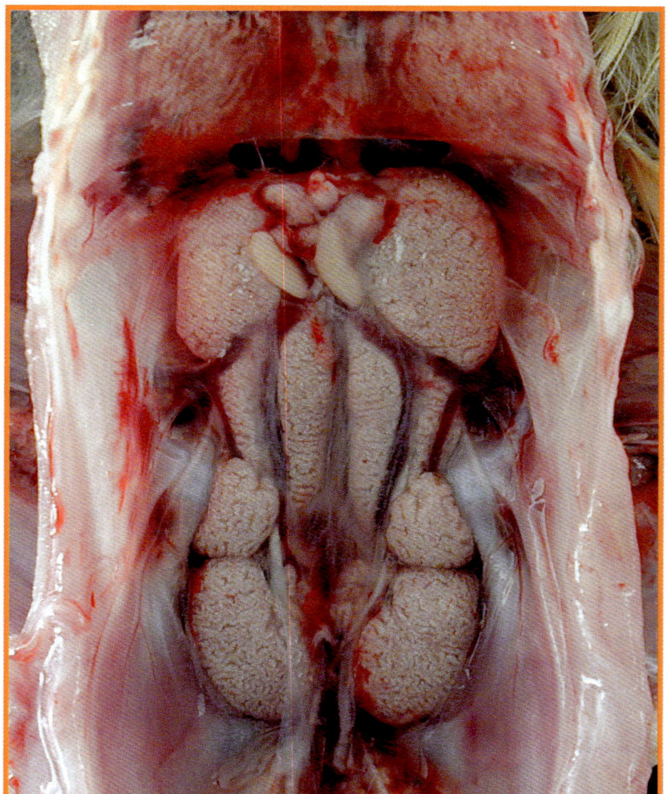

Fig. 105 | Nephritis with renal pallor and an accumulation of urates in a chicken suffering from acute IBD (Gumboro disease).

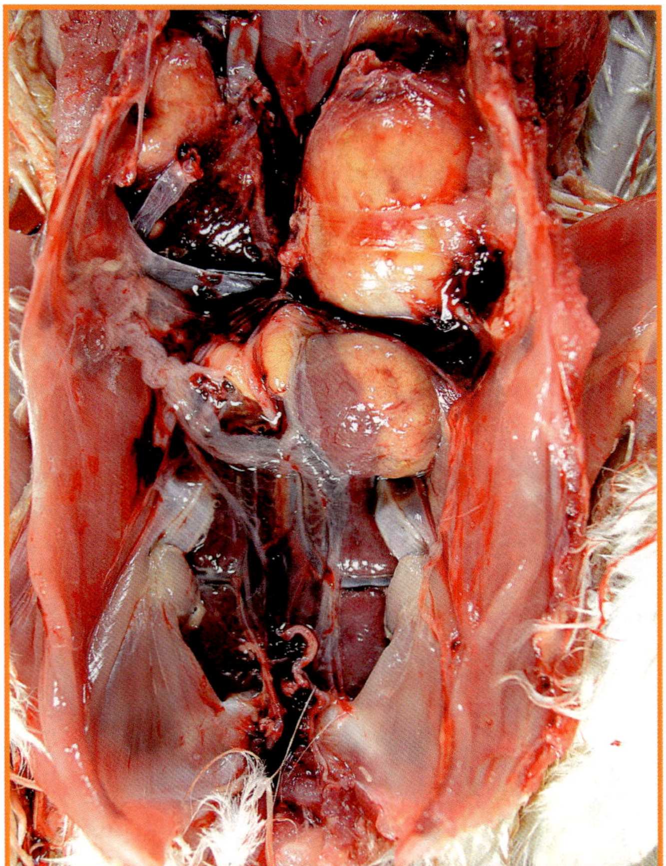

Fig. 106 | Nephritis and fungal granulomatous pneumonia.

- **Renal tumours:** the most common primary neoplasm is the nephroblastoma. However, lymphomas caused by viral infections (Marek's disease virus, lymphoid leukosis virus and myeloid reticuloendotheliosis virus) are also seen (fig. 107).

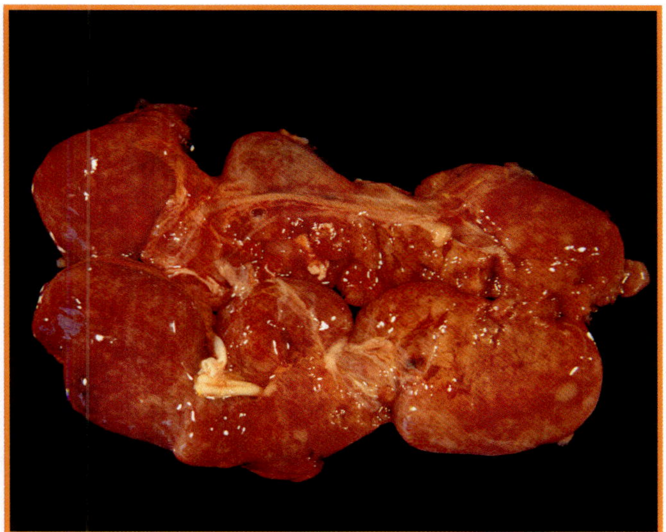

Fig. 107 | Renal lymphoma in a bird infected with lymphoid leukosis virus.

## Reproductive system

The evaluation and observation of lesions of the reproductive system is mainly carried out in laying birds or breeding birds, 18-20 weeks or older, once the system has developed to maturity. Throughout that time different stages of maturity of the reproductive system can be observed (fig. 108). The examination of the female reproductive system should include the **number and appearance of the ova**, the **size and appearance of the mucosa** of the oviduct, as well as the **presence of exudates** in the oviduct lumen.

The male reproductive system is simpler in terms of evaluation and observation of changes. It is essentially an examination of the **size and colour of the testes**.

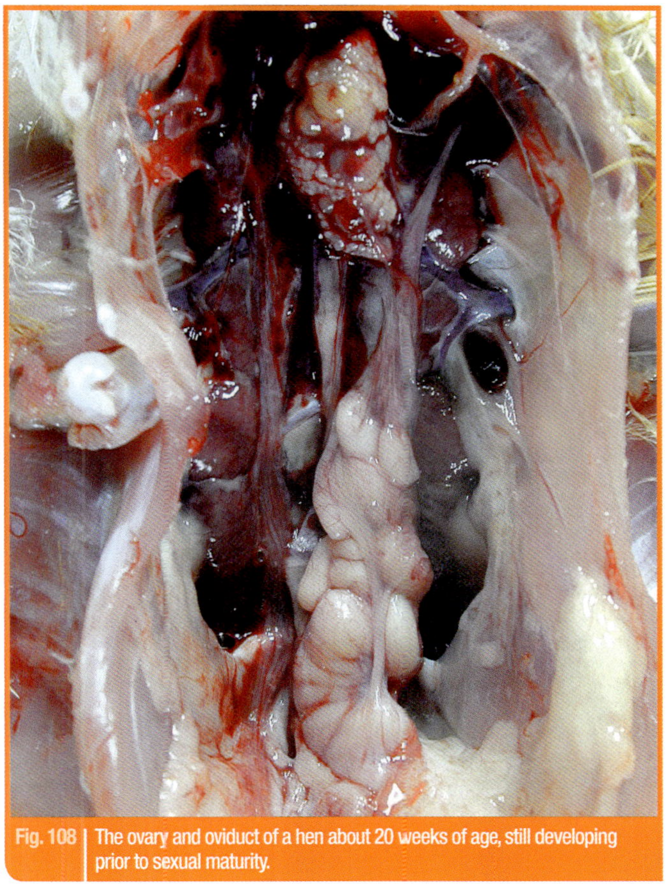

Fig. 108 | The ovary and oviduct of a hen about 20 weeks of age, still developing prior to sexual maturity.

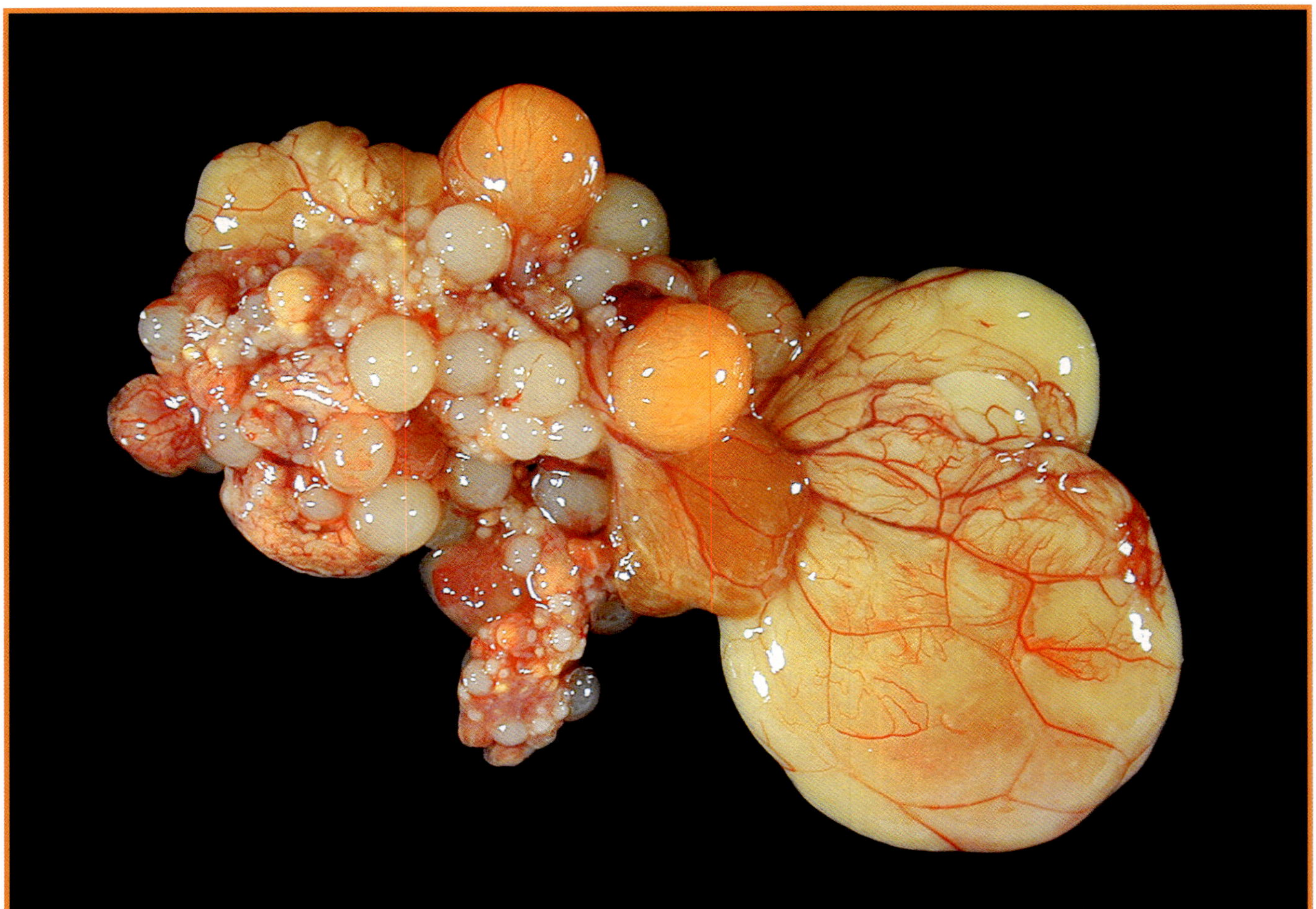

Fig. 109 | Ovarian regression. The ovary shown has virtually no large yellow follicle close to ovulation, but conversely it does have some atretic follicles.

The main changes to be observed in the female reproductive system are:

- **Ovarian regression:** it is associated with the hen reaching the end of the laying cycle or phase, or with various factors such as nutritional changes, infectious diseases, toxicity, hormonal manipulations or environmental factors which lead to cessation of ovulation. This process is called ovarian regression or atrophy (fig. 109). In the affected ovary new follicles will not develop and those present will suffer follicular atresia. **Ovarian follicular atresia** is the process whereby an ovule which has failed to ovulate, disappears and is reabsorbed. These follicles lose the characteristic shape and stiffness of developing follicles. The yolk they contain becomes more watery, less dense, and eventually they are reabsorbed into the bloodstream (fig. 110). This may be due to a physiological process since not all developing ova arrive to ovulation, or, due to a pathological process that induces ovarian regression.

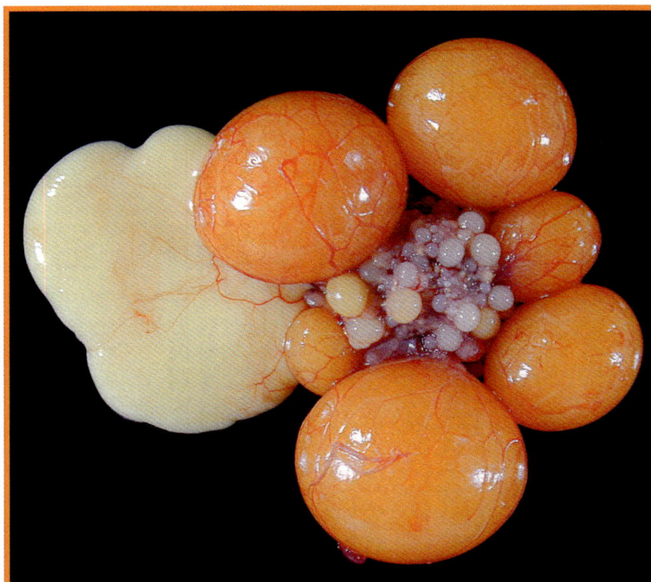

Fig. 110 | Functional ovary of a 35-week-old hen. Six large yellow follicles are seen alongside one atretic follicle. This has lost its turgor and displays a paler colour.

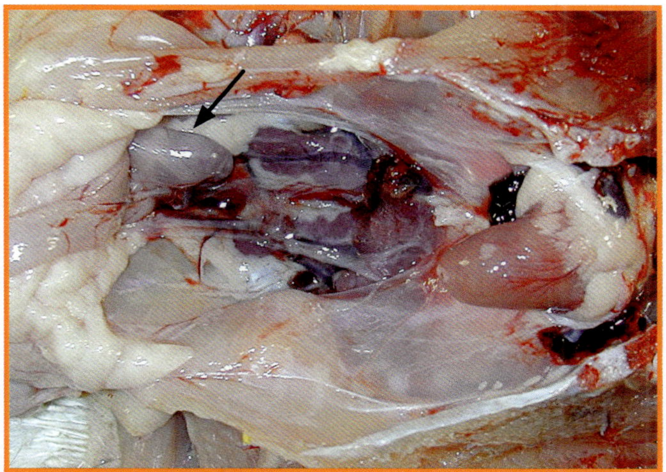
Fig. 111 | A persistent right oviduct in a bird (arrow). A cyst with clear fluid can be seen in the region to the right of the cloaca.

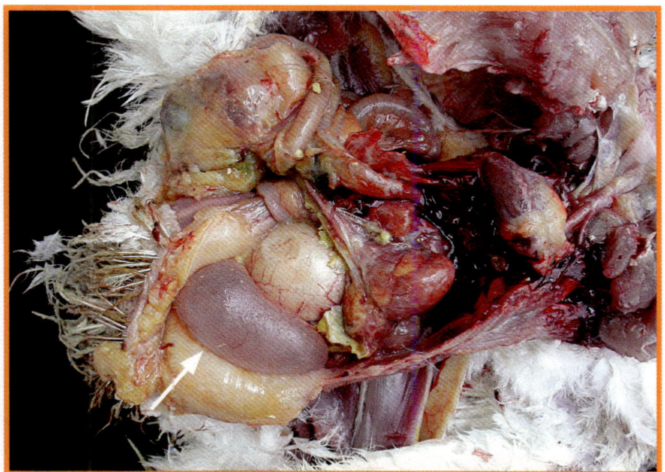
Fig. 112 | Coelomic cavity of a 40-week-old chicken with a persistent right oviduct (arrow). A fluid-filled diverticulum in the caudal region can also be seen.

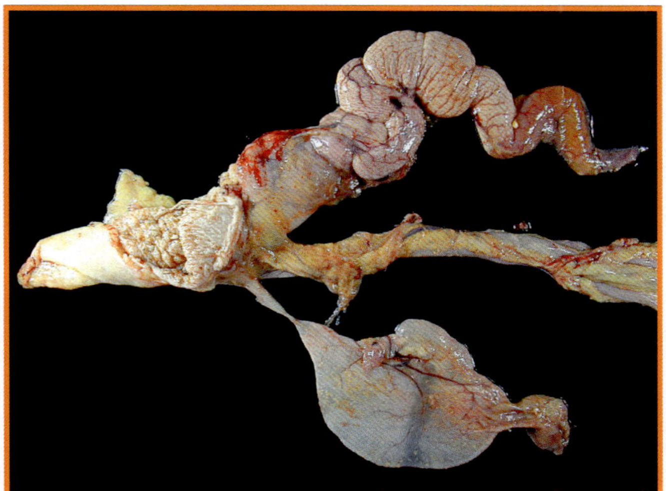
Fig. 113 | Persistent right oviduct and a functional left oviduct.

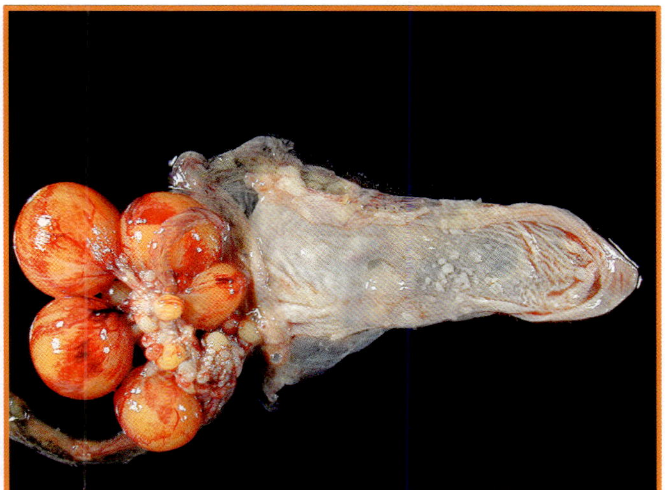
Fig. 114 | Hypoplastic oviduct occluded in the caudal region.

- **Persistent right oviduct:** in some cases the right-side ovary and oviduct may not disappear but accumulate clear liquid which forms a cyst on the right side of the cloaca. This persistent or cystic right oviduct is observed in birds that have not yet reached sexual maturity (fig. 111), as well as in adult birds (figs. 112 and 113).
- **Oviduct hypoplasia:** it is an abnormality characterised by an incomplete development of the oviduct. Macroscopically, a shorter oviduct is seen, and also in some cases, the end of the lumen becomes occluded (figs. 114 and 115). This may be due to genetic causes or early infections before the bird reaches sexual maturity (e.g., infectious bronchitis virus).

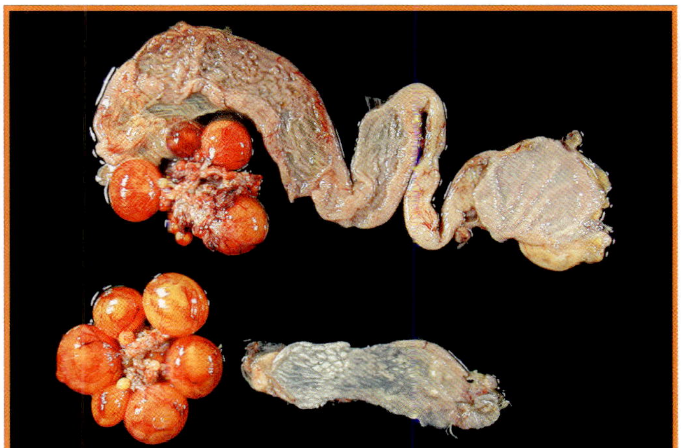
Fig. 115 | Oviduct hypoplasia. The top part of the image shows a normal oviduct, while underneath is a shorter oviduct. Here it is impossible to distinguish the different regions.

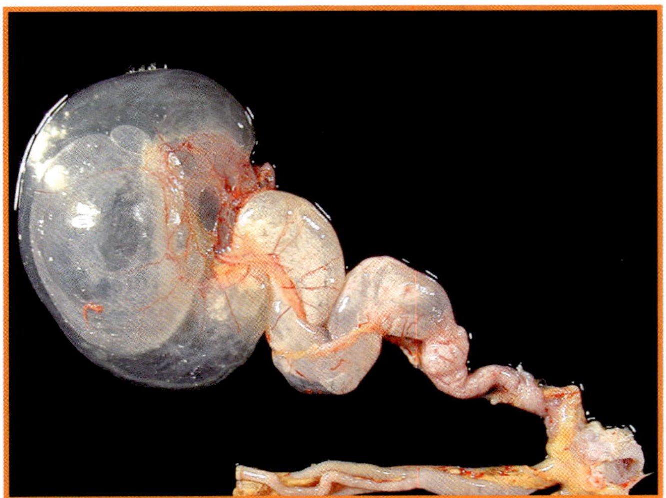

Fig. 116 | A cystic oviduct of a hen. The accumulation of clear fluid in the oviduct lumen forming cysts in the cranial region of the infundibulum is shown.

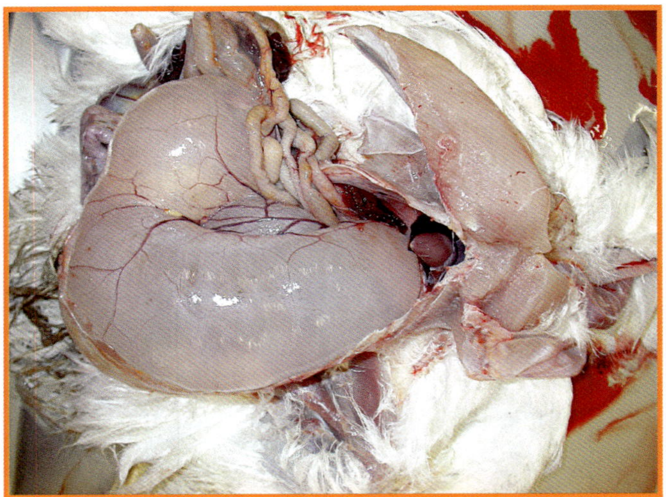

Fig. 117 | A cystic oviduct that occupies a large part of the chicken's coelomic cavity.

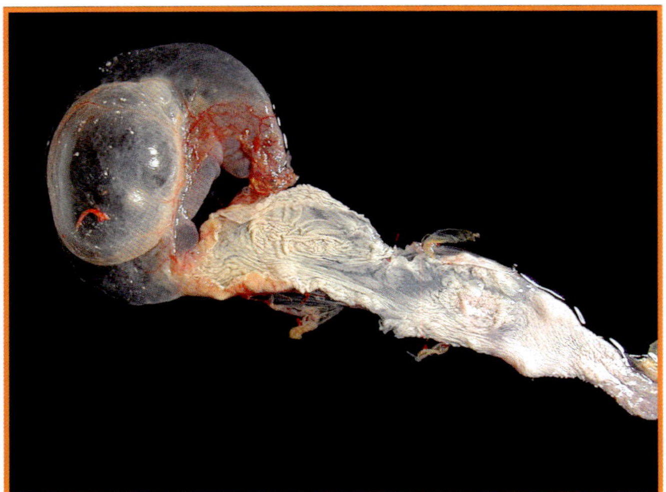

Fig. 118 | A cystic oviduct with areas where the oviduct wall is much thinner than normal with very few folds.

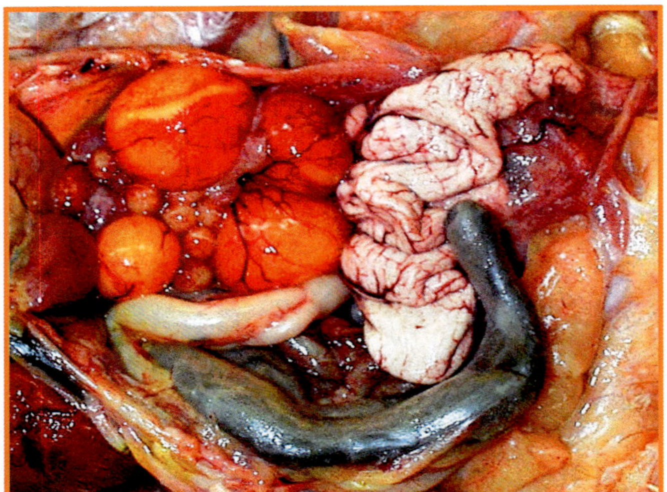

Fig. 119 | Oophoritis with significant congestion of the ova.

- **Hydropic or cystic oviduct:** in some cases, not only is an incomplete oviduct development observed, but also fluid builds up inside the oviduct resulting in cysts (fig. 116). If a large quantity of fluid accumulates, cysts with clear fluid will be found occupying part of the coelomic cavity (fig. 117). On opening the affected oviducts, an alteration in the mucosa is seen (fig. 118). It is associated to the same causes as hypoplasia of the oviduct.
- **Oophoritis (ovaritis):** it is the inflammation of the ovary usually associated with bacterial infections (e.g., *Salmonella, E. coli*). The affected ovary shows congestion, and the affected follicles lose their shape and often have a haemorrhagic appearance (fig. 119).
- **Salpingitis:** when the inflammation affects the oviduct it is called salpingitis and it is a major cause of egg production loss and lower egg quality. It can be caused by bacterial or viral infections. Generally, salpingitis due to bacterial infection is more exudative with fibrin masses forming in the oviduct lumen (fig. 120), and in some situations, yolk and egg remains (fig. 121). By contrast, in virus associated

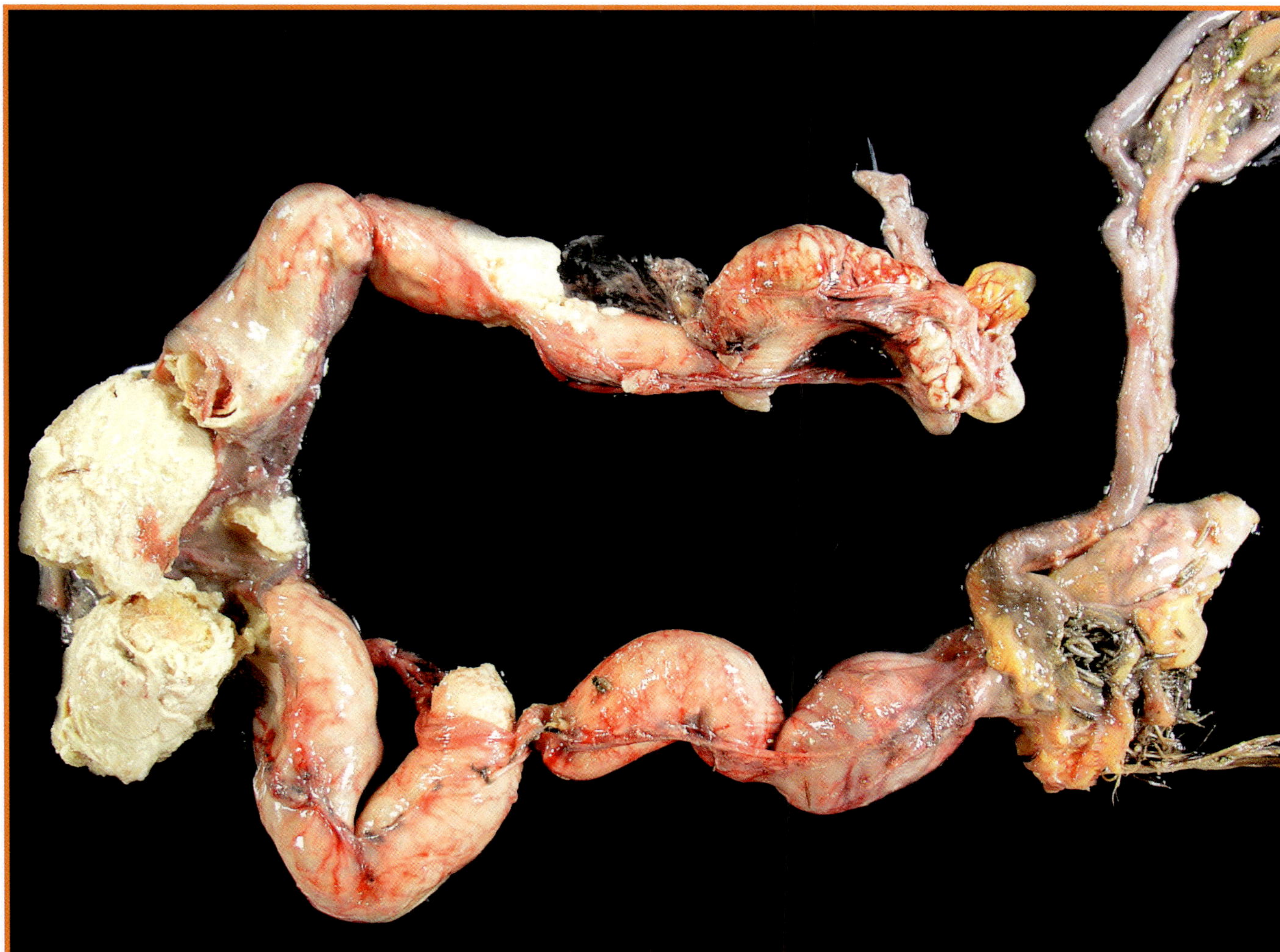

Fig. 120 | Fibrinous salpingitis with caseous material that has taken the tubular shape of the oviduct.

salpingitis, oedema and congestion of the oviduct mucosa are observed, as well as cloudy or gelatinous exudate in some cases, but large deposits of fibrin are not seen. The affected region of the oviduct varies according to the virus which has infected the bird. This, in turn, alters one part or another of the egg in formation. For example, strains of the infectious bronchitis virus able to replicate in the oviduct do so in the magnum, the region where the albumen is formed. This results in the eggs forming with altered and irregular albumen, and the shell is then deposited irregularly,

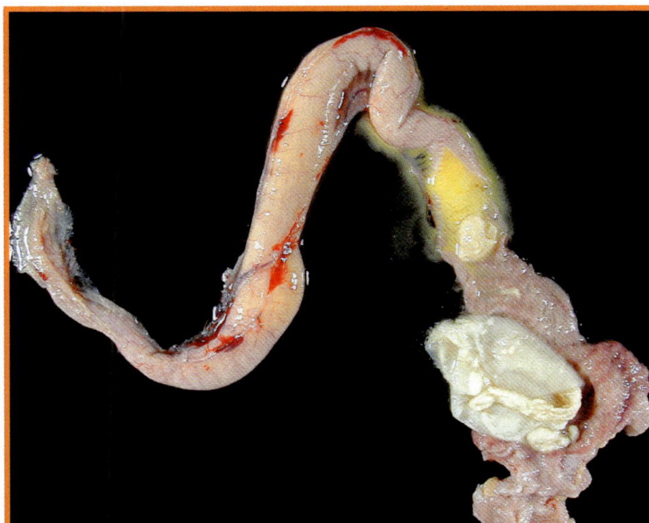

Fig. 121 | Fibrinous salpingitis with remains of an egg in formation, cloudy white exudates and caseous material in the lumina of the isthmus and uterus.

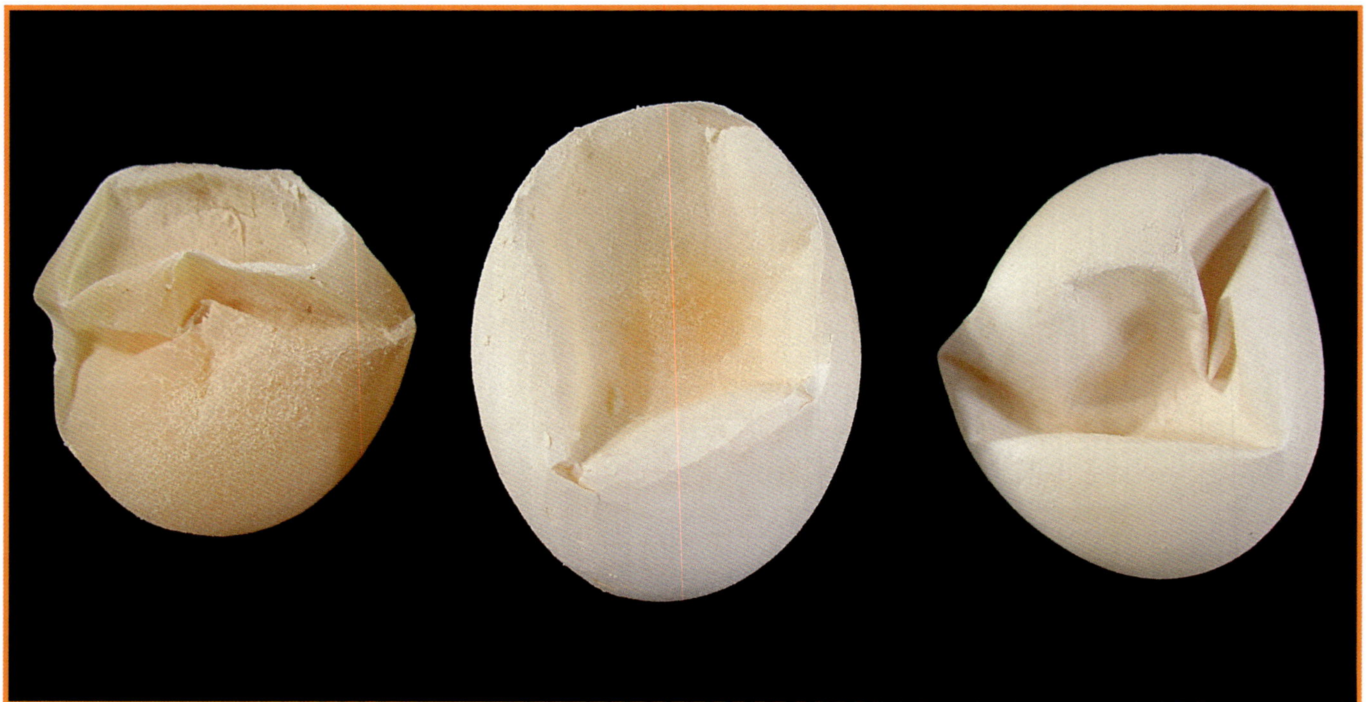

Fig. 122 | Soft-shell eggs. The shell deposition of the eggs has not been produced correctly and therefore the shell is much thinner.

producing rough-shelled eggs. In contrast, the avian adenovirus (egg drop syndrome) replicates in the uterus, altering the deposition of the egg shell and resulting in soft-shell eggs (fig. 122).

- **Peritonitis caused by intra-abdominal ovulation or laying:** it is the inflammation of the coelomic cavity caused by ovulated follicles falling into the cavity instead of the oviduct. A gross observation finds fibrinous exudate together with traces of yolk or egg in the serous membranes of the coelomic cavity (fig. 123). This may be due to various causes such as malformations of the oviduct (hypoplastic oviducts with occluded entry) or mobility of the oviduct. Eggs have also been found in the coelomic cavity due to retroperistalsic movements of the oviduct. As with intra-abdominal ovulation, this too may lead to peritonitis.
- **Tumours:** different types of tumours may be seen in the female reproductive system. Viral lymphomas (Marek's disease virus, lymphoid leukosis virus and myeloid reticuloendotheliosis virus) normally affect the ovary. In addition, gonadal tumours (granulosa cells), germ cell tumours (seminomas in males and dysgerminomas in females), epithelial cell tumours (adenomas and adenocarcinomas) and mesenchymal tumours (leiomyoma) may be found. Leiomyomas, adenomas and adenocarcinomas are the most common neoplasms in the chicken's reproductive system and are easy to observe in old hens.

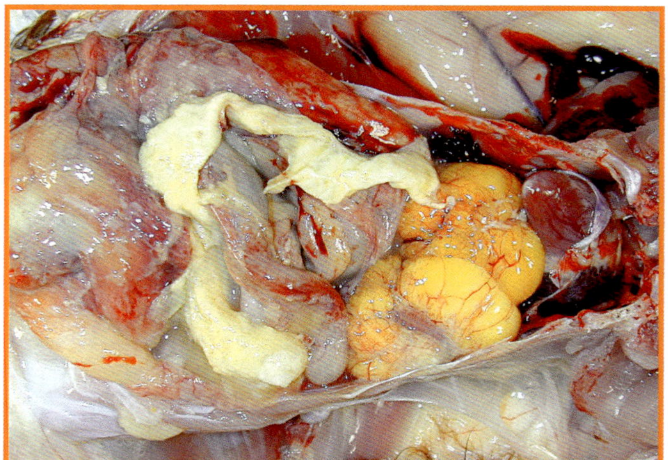

Fig. 123 | Peritonitis with large amounts of fibrinous exudate and traces of yolk seen both in the coelomic cavity and on the serous membrane of the cavity organs.

- **Orchitis:** it is an inflammation of the testes usually accompanied by inflammation of the epididymis (epididymo-orchitis). It is usually associated with bacterial infections (*E. coli*, *Pasteurella*, *Salmonella*), and the testes appear enlarged, irregular, with significant vascularisation and areas of discoloration.

# Musculoskeletal system

Included in this section are the lesions affecting the bones, the muscles and the joints. An important comment to begin with is the similarity between the clinical symptoms associated with musculoskeletal lesions in birds, and those observed in animals affected by central or peripheral nervous system disorders (fig. 124). Therefore in these clinical cases, it is advisable to perform both macroscopic and microscopic evaluations on all the organs that may be involved (muscles, bones, joints, central and peripheral nervous system) to determine the origin of the symptoms.

## Bones

As already mentioned, in any necropsy it is advisable to inspect the condition of the bones. An external evaluation, especially of the leg bones, is recommended to detect possible deformities and also determine the degree of calcification of the bone. Normally, the **degree of calcification** is evaluated by extracting the femur or the tibiotarsus and applying pressure to try to break it in half. If the bone bends, but does not break, it is very indicative of a calcification problem. In this case, it would be necessary to take samples of the metaphysis or growth plate for microscopic evaluation. Some of the major pathological processes that affect the bone are:

- **Spondylolisthesis:** it is a defect in the development of the sixth thoracic vertebra causing a rotation of the vertebral body, pressure on the spinal cord and paralysis of the legs. The affected birds "sit" on their own legs (fig. 125). At necropsy, a thickening of the spine's ventral region at the affected vertebra level can be observed (fig. 126).
- **Bone deformities of the extremities:** there are multiple disorders with lameness and gross alterations associated with the bones of the extremities including reduction in the length of the bones (e.g., perosis or chondrodystrophy), rotation of the shafts (e.g., rotation of the tibia) or the epiphyses of the bones (e.g., varus-valgus deformity). In general, these processes are rare, with poorly defined aetiology, which probably involve nutritional (deficiencies of vitamins or minerals), metabolic or genetic factors (figs. 127 and 128).

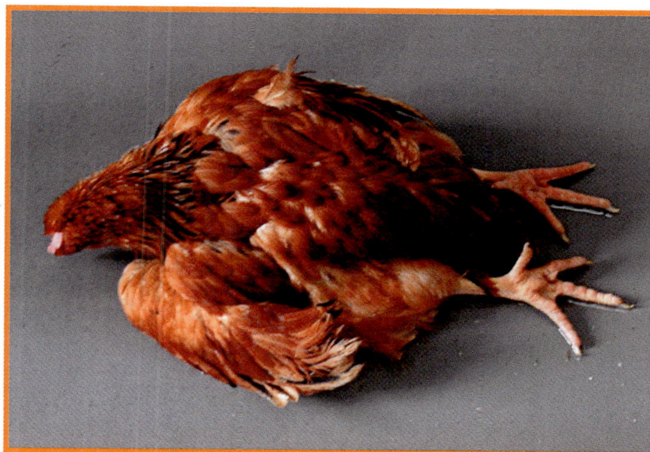

Fig. 124 | A prostrate bird with leg paralysis. An animal with toxic myopathy caused by excess monensin in the feed. These symptoms, however, could be observed in other processes which affect the nervous system or the bones.

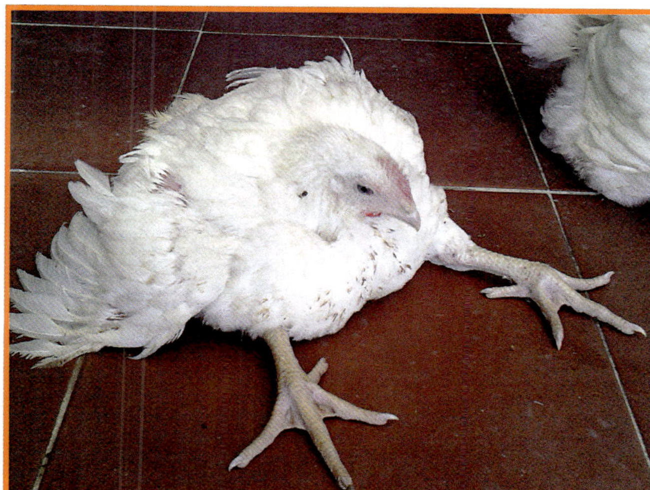

Fig. 125 | A bird affected by spondylolisthesis "sitting" on its own legs.

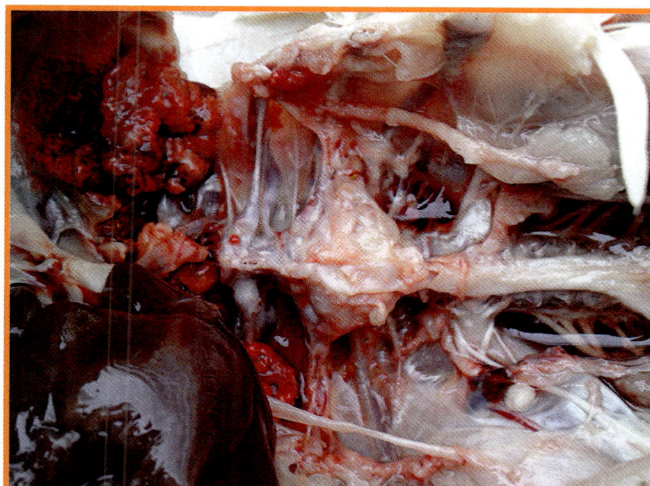

Fig. 126 | Spondylolisthesis. The ventral part of the spine shows a focal thickening in the spine's ventral region at the level of the sixth thoracic vertebra.

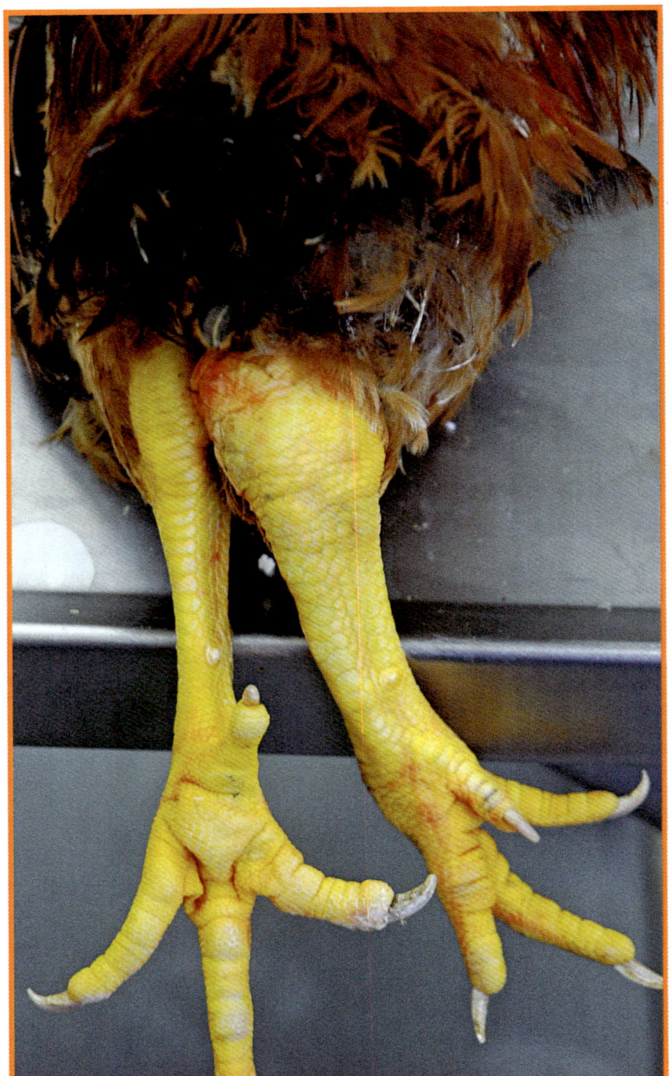

Fig. 127 | Varus-valgus deformation and an epiphysis rotation of the distal end of the right tibiotarsus.

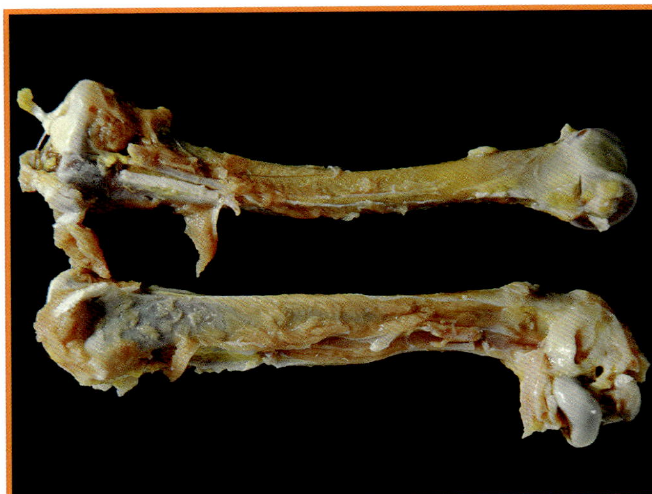

Fig. 128 | A tibiotarsus varus-valgus deformity, with an epiphysis rotation of the distal end of the right tibiotarsus.

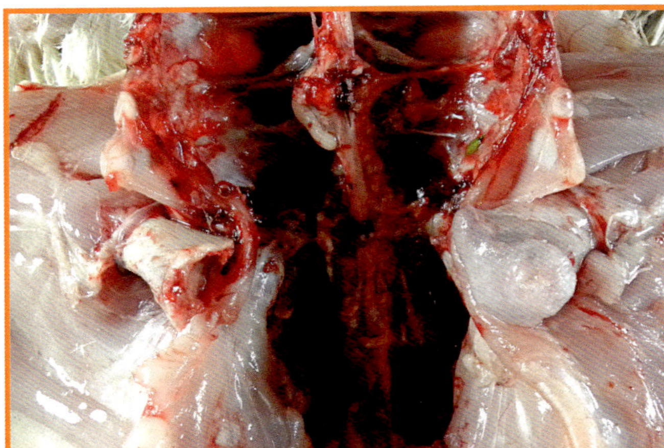

Fig. 129 | Femur heads. The left femur shows necrosis and osteomyelitis with significant bone loss, whereas the right femur only presents articular cartilage loss which is possibly artefactual.

- **Necrosis of the femoral head:** it is a relatively common lesion, but its clinical diagnosis requires a careful evaluation of the affected bone. There are alterations which should not be considered as a lesion, such as the separation of the articular cartilage of the femoral head caused by the tensile force used at necropsy to dismantle the coxofemoral joint (fig. 129). It is therefore advisable to evaluate the femoral head in several different animals from the batch and consider the clinical signs. The main lesion to observe is the rupture of the femoral head often accompanied by a significant loss of bone tissue (figs. 129 and 130). In birds, this injury may be associated with bacterial infections, which are usually systemic.

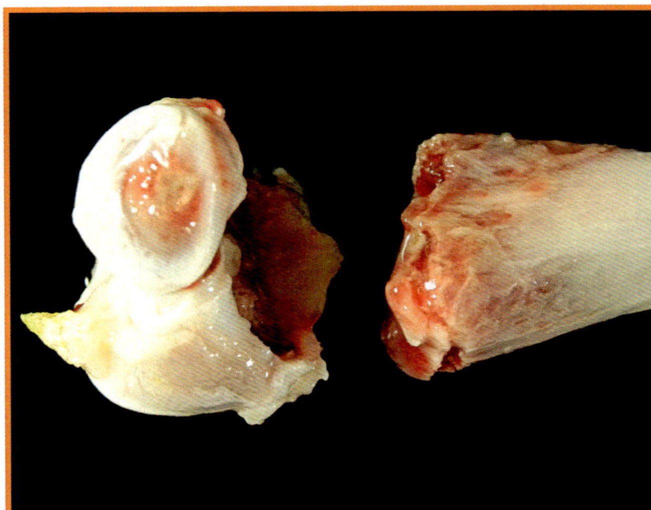

Fig. 130 | Rupture (epiphysiolysis) of the femoral head.

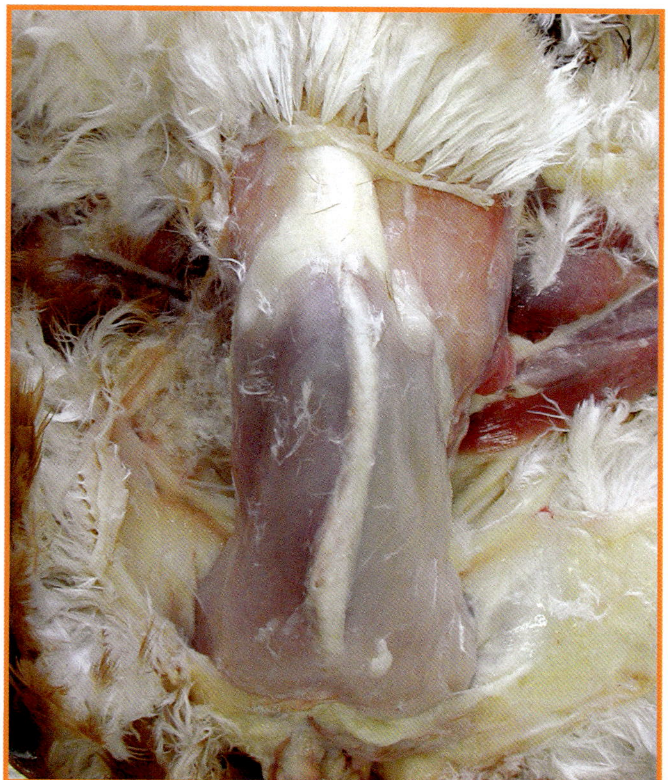

Fig. 131 | A laying hen displaying rickets with deformation of the keel and pectoral muscle atrophy.

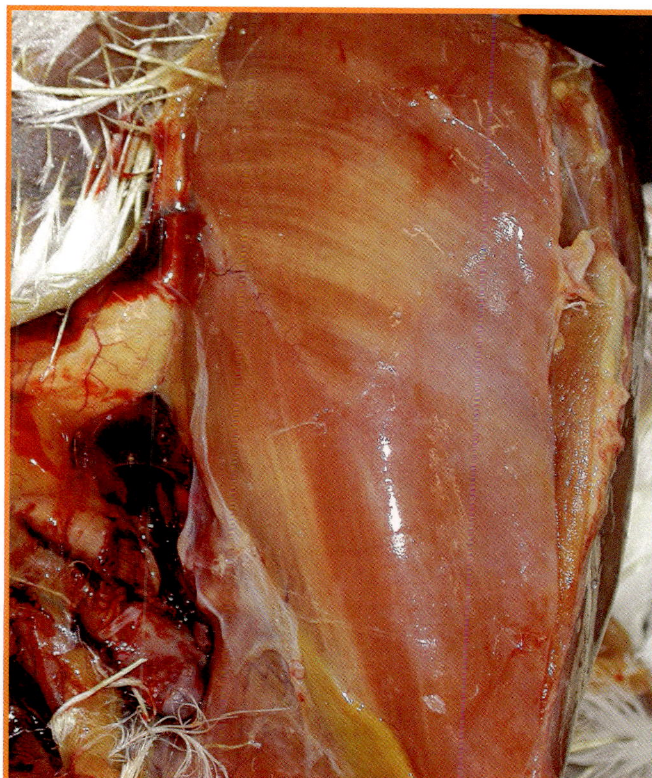

Fig. 132 | Nutritional myopathy characterised by paler coloration bands in the pectoral muscle

- **Rickets:** the deficits of calcium, phosphorus or vitamin D can cause bone alterations. It is usually seen in chicks or laying hens, and is associated with general weakness and prostration. At necropsy, a decrease in bone consistency, such as bending the bones or the peak without breaking, is normally detected. In severe cases the keel (fig. 131) and the rachitic rosary (thickening of the costochondral joints) may be deformed.
- **Tibial dyschondroplasia:** the presence of an abnormal mass of whitish cartilage in the proximal tibial epiphysis which causes lameness especially in broiler chickens, turkeys and ducks.

## Muscles

The examination of the animal's muscles is primarily focused on the evaluation of **volume** and **coloration**. Even so, there are not many pathological processes with gross visible lesions in the muscles. The major pathological processes that affect this tissue are:

- **Muscle atrophy:** it is a decrease in the normal muscle volume, and the examination is based on the appearance of the pectoral muscles. Anorexia and progressive loss of body weight are chronic syndromes. It should be highlighted that when assessing an animal's muscle volume, the age and stock must be taken into account.
- **Nutritional or toxic myopathy:** these two disorders, despite having a very different aetiology, have very similar gross and microscopic lesions. A gross examination shows paler coloured, including yellow, bands in the muscles (fig. 132) which correspond to areas of segmental necrosis of the muscle fibres (fig. 133). It should be noted that gross lesions are not always observed in the affected animals, although microscopic lesions exist. Therefore, if either of these disorders is suspected, then muscle samples must be taken for histological analysis. The main aetiology of nutritional myopathy is a deficiency of antioxidants (vitamin E and selenium), while toxic myopathy is usually caused by an excess of ionophore antibiotics in animal feed.
- **Green Muscle Disease:** it is a greenish coloration of the deep pectoral muscle due to ischemic necrosis (fig. 134). It is seen in heavy stock, mainly broiler and turkey.

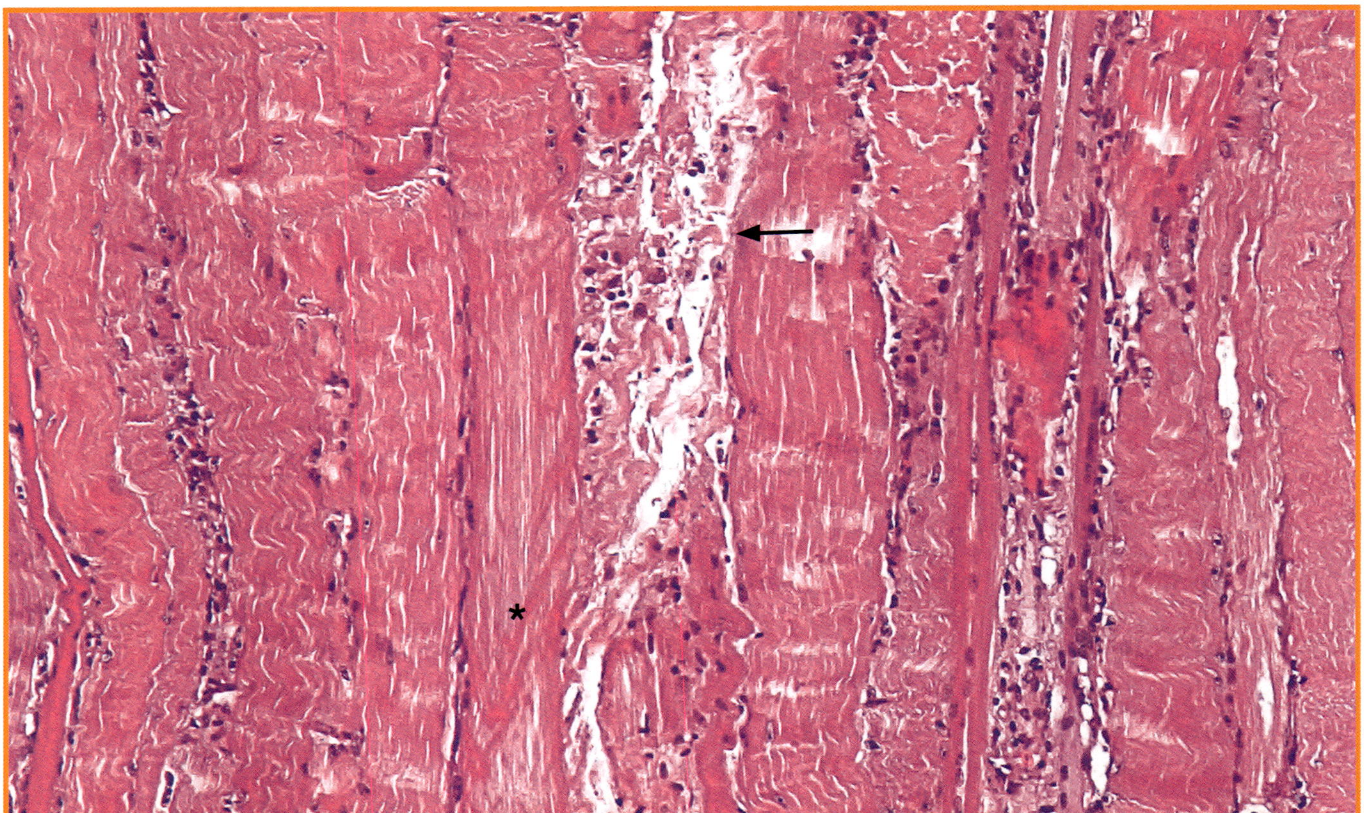

Fig. 133 | Microscopic image of the musculature of an animal affected by toxic myopathy, which shows hyalinization and fragmentation of muscle fibres (arrow). The asterisk shows a non-affected muscle fibre.

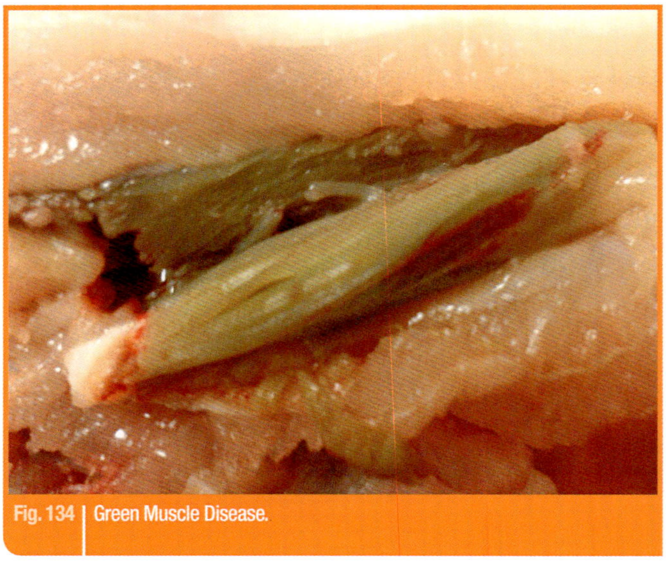

Fig. 134 | Green Muscle Disease.

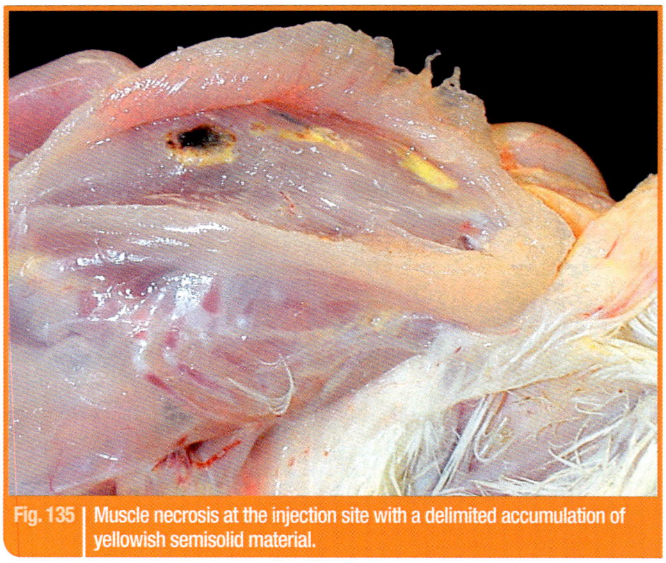

Fig. 135 | Muscle necrosis at the injection site with a delimited accumulation of yellowish semisolid material.

- **Muscle necrosis at the injection site:** the injection of antibiotics or adjuvant vaccines can cause necrosis and granulomatous inflammation at the injection site, seen as a delimited whitish or yellowish cluster of semisolid consistency (fig. 135), or as an area of muscle discoloration (fig. 136).
- **Muscle haemorrhages:** it is not a specific lesion, but it may be seen associated with trauma or infections such as IBD (Gumboro disease, fig. 137).

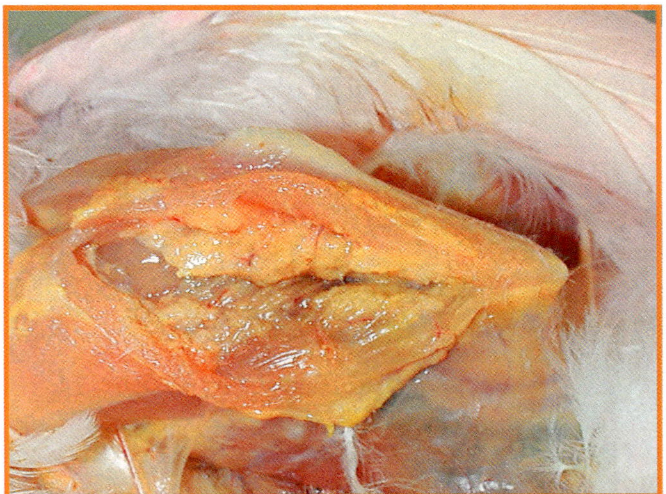

Fig. 136 | Muscle necrosis at the injection site. Large area of muscle discoloration.

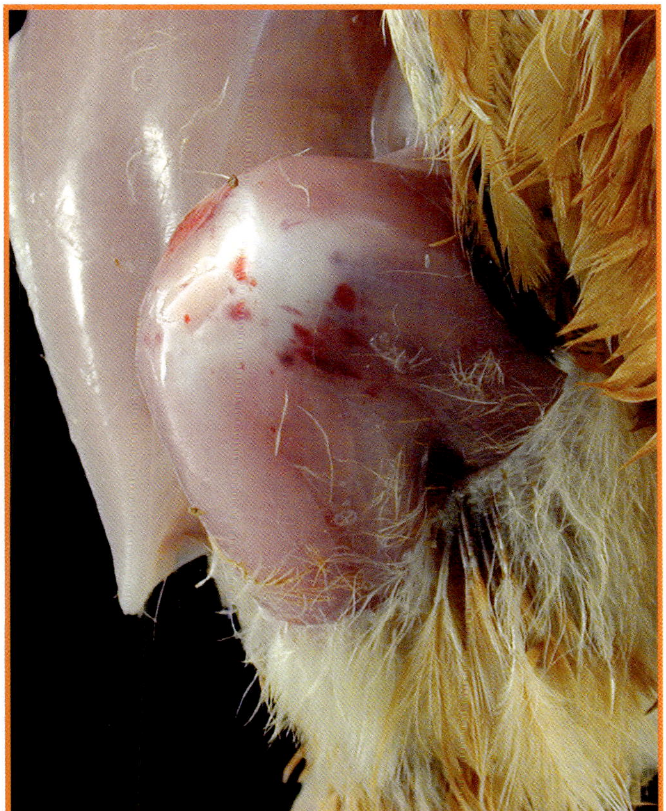

Fig. 137 | Muscle haemorrhage in the thigh of a bird affected by IBD (Gumboro disease).

## Joints and tendons

The most important process which can be observed in the joints and tendons is inflammation or arthritis. This is usually associated with swelling of the affected joint which is then visible externally (fig. 138) and, once sectioned, purulent exudate will be present in the joint cavity. Erosions can also be seen on the surface of articular cartilage, and thickening of the inside of the joint capsule if chronic. The main articular processes are:

- **Fibrinopurulent arthritis:** it is characterised by the presence of abundant fibrinopurulent exudate in the joint cavity (fig. 139). It is normally associated to bacterial septicaemia (*Staphylococcus aureus*, *Escherichia coli, Salmonella* spp., etc.) or to *Mycoplasma synoviae* infection.
- **Tenosynovitis:** it is an extensive inflammation of the gastrocnemius tendon region, above the tarsometatarsal joint, together with oedema and haemorrhage (fig. 140) and may affect the digital flexor and extensor tendons. This may lead to rupture of the affected tendons (fig. 141). The location of the lesion is mainly at the tendon sheath as seen in the cross-section of the tendons. In chronic cases, tendon fibrosis may be observed. In general, tendon lesions are not

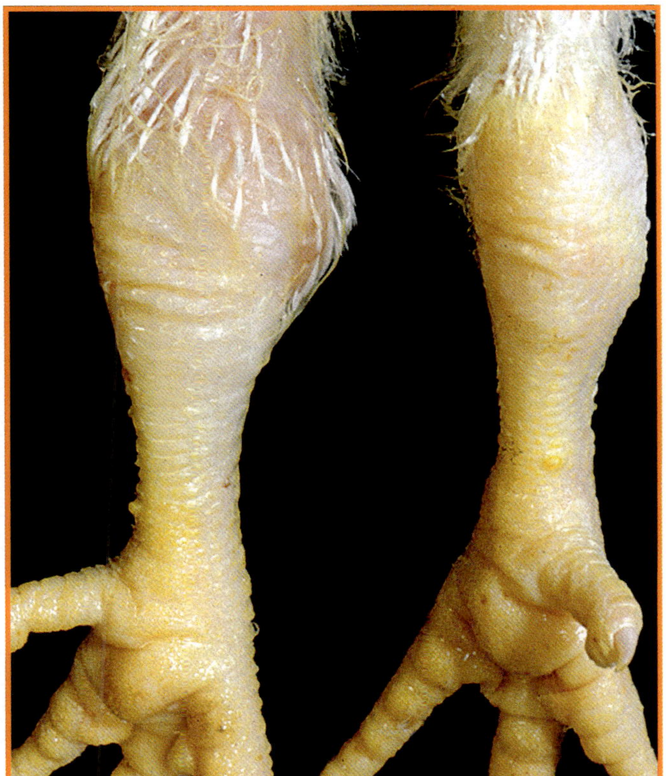

Fig. 138 | Unilateral swelling of the tibiometatarsal joint in an animal affected by arthritis.

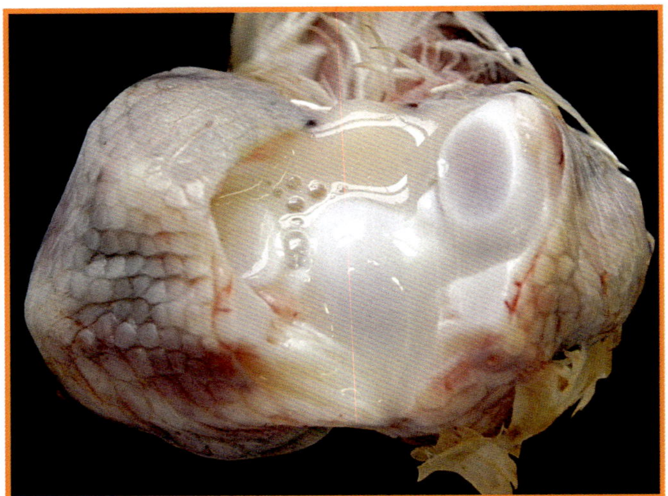

Fig. 139 | Purulent arthritis due to *S. aureus*. The joint cavity has abundant purulent exudate.

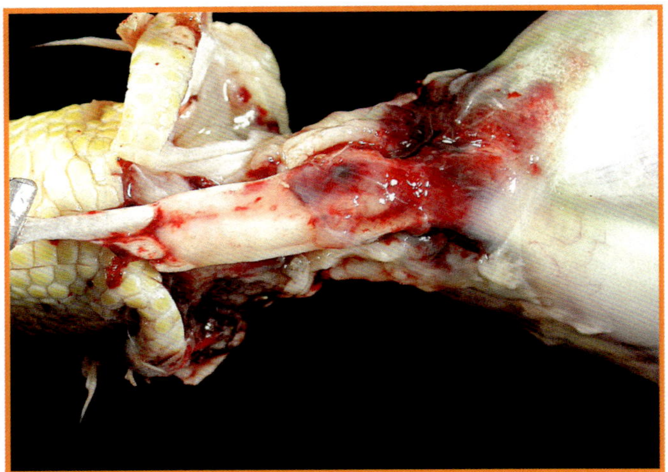

Fig. 140 | Viral tenosynovitis characterised by intense oedema and haemorrhage in the gastrocnemius tendon sheath, above the tarsometatarsal joint.

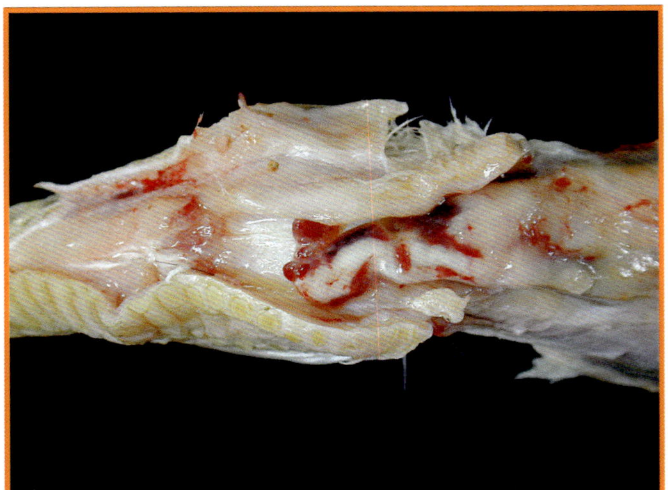

Fig. 141 | Rupture of the gastrocnemius tendon in a case of tenosynovitis virus.

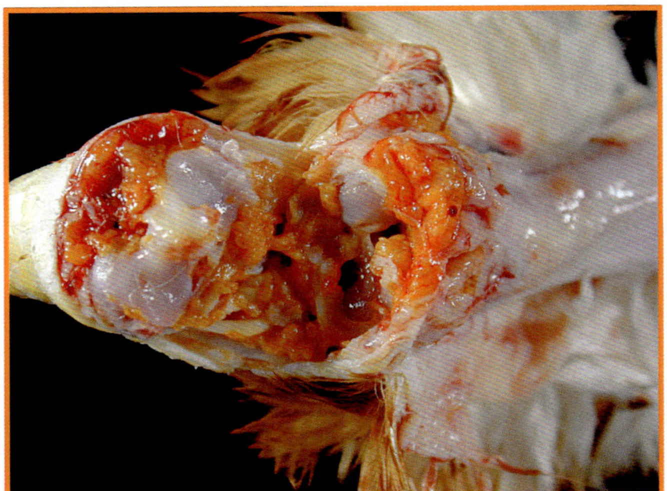

Fig. 142 | Amyloid arthropathy with an accumulation of orange coloured material (amyloid) on the inside of the joint capsule and articular cartilage erosions.

associated with changes found in the joint cavity. This process is caused by an avian reoviral infection.

- **Amyloid arthropathy:** it is characterised by an over-filled joint capsule with clusters of orange-coloured amyloid material (fig. 142). Amyloid is composed of serum proteins deposited in various organs including joints during a chronic infection. This lesion is associated with chronic bacterial infections, the most frequent being *Enterococcus faecalis*, but it may also be caused by other bacterial pathogens such as *Salmonella* spp., *Mycoplasma* spp., etc. It is a pathological process which appears more often in laying hens.
- **Articular gout:** it is a deposit of uric acid crystals identified as white granular material in the joint. It is normally associated with impaired renal function.

# Nervous system

This section includes the lesions which affect the nervous system. The evaluation of the nervous system should include an examination of the peripheral nerves, the sciatic nerve and the central nervous system including the brain and the spinal cord. Unlike other systems or apparatus, the alterations in the nervous system induce fairly indicative clinical signs such as incoordination, pedalling movements, paralysis or opisthotonos (fig. 143). However, it should be remembered that in the moments before death, or in cases of diseases affecting the musculoskeletal system, the animal may show similar clinical signs.

In most cases, although a medical condition of the nervous system is evident, the macroscopic evaluation of both the peripheral nerves as well as the central nervous system is often unproductive as it is difficult to observe gross lesions. Even so, if an alteration of the nervous system is suspected, it is necessary to conduct a histopathological study which will probably show the presence of histological lesions in the tissues. For this reason, most images included in this chapter show the histological lesions observed in each case.

## Central nervous system

The main lesions found in the central nervous system are detailed below:

- **Haemorrhages:** cerebral haemorrhages are not frequent, and they may be primarily due to traumatic head injury or secondary due to infectious processes or necrosis.
- **Encephalomalacia:** it is **necrosis** of the nervous tissue of the brain. Gross observation of this lesion is difficult. It is only possible to observe whitish areas and haemorrhages on the brain surface in very severe cases. By contrast, microscopic examination shows very evident lesions such as large areas of spongiosis (fig. 144), thrombi in the blood vessels (fig. 145) and haemorrhages. This lesion is primarily associated with vitamin E and selenium deficiency in young birds or salt poisoning. When the lesion is located in the optic lobes it may be associated with a septicaemia due to *Enterococcus hirae*. When necrosis occurs in the spinal cord nervous tissue, the lesion is known as **myelomalacia**.

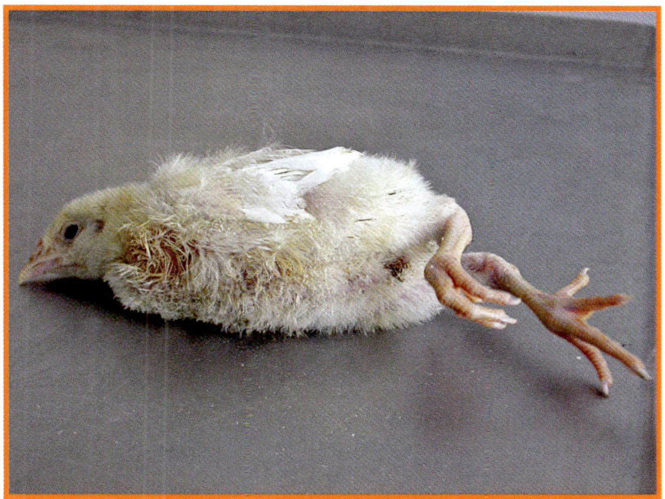

Fig. 143 | An animal with incoordination and pedal movements.

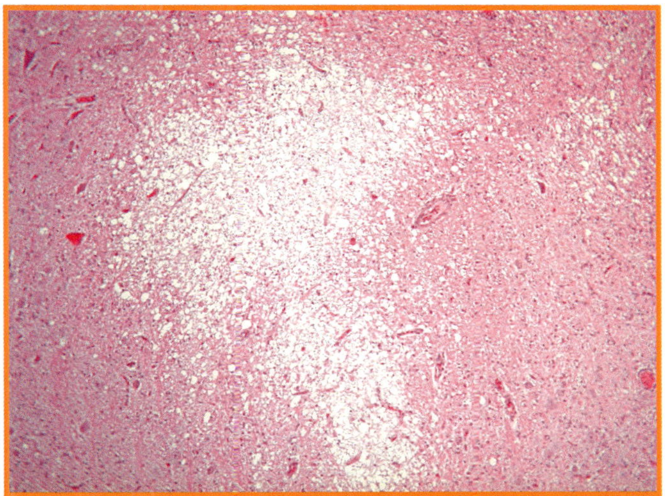

Fig. 144 | Microscopic image of encephalomalacia, showing an extensive area of malacia. H&E stain.

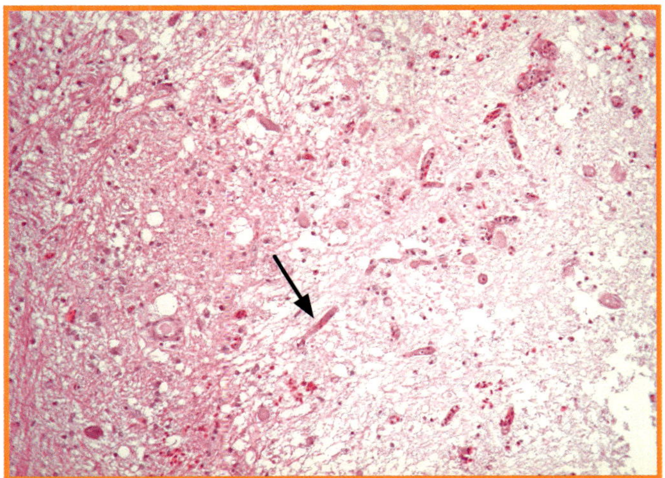

Fig. 145 | Microscopic image of a case of encephalomalacia, showing thrombi (arrow) in the vessels located in the malacia area. H&E stain.

- **Central nervous system inflammation:** the nomenclature of inflammation in the nervous system depends on the regions affected. The inflammation may affect the brain (encephalitis), the meninges (meningitis) or the spinal cord (myelitis). If the inflammation is seen in more than one region, this terminology can be combined resulting in encephalomyelitis, meningoencephalitis, or meningoencephalomyelitis. In addition, depending on the nature of the inflammatory infiltrate, the inflammation may be described as non-suppurative (mononuclear cell infiltration), suppurative (heterophil infiltration) or granulomatous. An inflammation of the nervous system in birds results primarily from infectious causes:
  - **Virus.** Although lesions are not usually seen, some viral infections may cause brain congestion (fig. 146). Microscopically, however, they produce a non-purulent encephalitis with gliosis, neuronal degeneration and perivascular cuffing (fig. 147). The main viruses which cause brain lesions are the highly pathogenic avian influenza virus and the neurotropic velogenic Newcastle virus. If a nervous disorder is seen in chicks younger than 6 weeks old, then avian encephalomyelitis virus must be discarded. This virus may infect adult birds, but in these cases the infection is often subclinical. Microscopically, the presence of perivascular cuffing, neuronal chromatolysis (fig. 148) and multifocal microgliosis in the Purkinje cell layer is pathognomonic. Finally, an infection of very virulent Marek's disease virus (vvMDV; *very virulent*) or extremely virulent (vv+MDV; *very virulent plus*) Marek's disease virus strains may induce acute transient paralysis or flaccid neck paralysis. The clinical signs are highly indicative, as the paralysis prevents the animal from keeping the neck upright (fig. 149). This paralysis is transient, unlike the cases of botulism, and birds recover in 48-72 hours if they have access to water and feed. A diagnosis confirmation is obtained by a histopathological study of the brain, which shows vasculitis.
  - **Bacteria.** A bacterial infection of the brain is uncommon and includes suppurative or granulomatous encephalitis. It originates either in septicaemia, in which the bacteria also reaches the central nervous system (e.g., *Salmonella* spp., *E. coli*, *Staphylococcus* spp., *Streptococcus* spp., *Pseudomonas* spp. o *Pasteurella* spp.), or in otitis media/internal, in which the infection spreads to the brain (e.g., *Pasteurella* spp.,

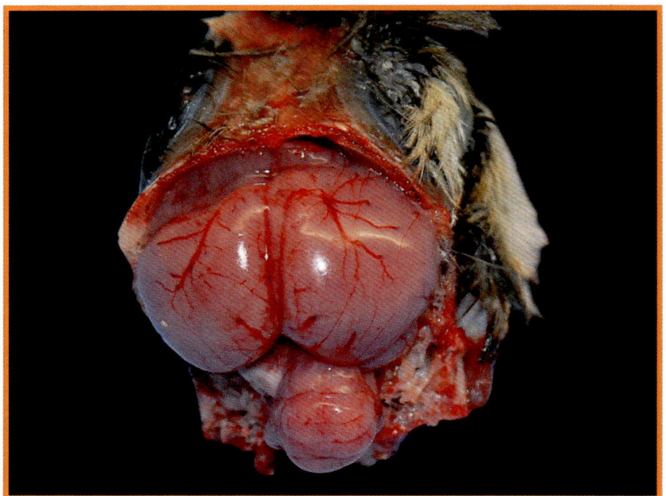
Fig. 146 | Brain congestion in a partridge affected by highly pathogenic avian influenza.

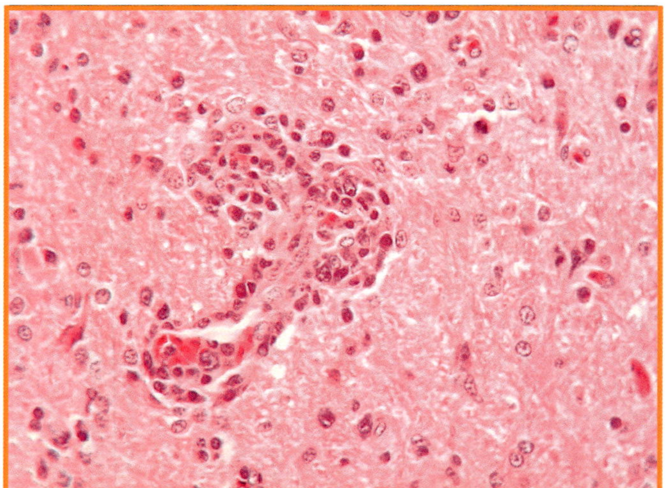
Fig. 147 | Microscopic image of avian encephalomalacia, showing perivascular cuffing H&E stain.

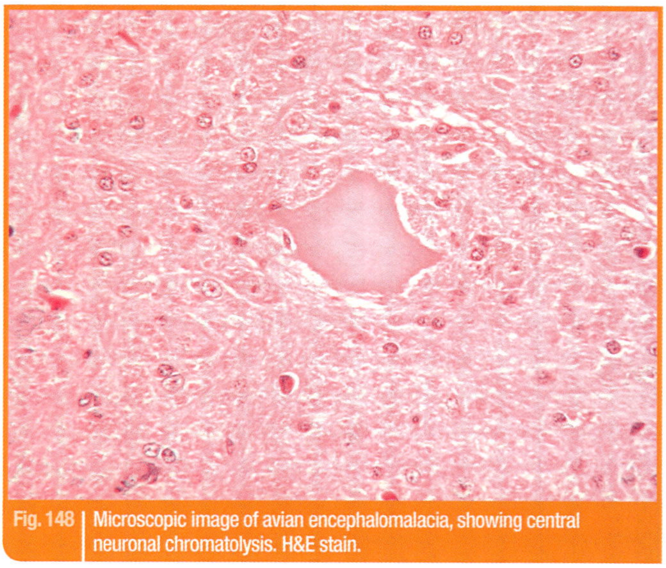
Fig. 148 | Microscopic image of avian encephalomalacia, showing central neuronal chromatolysis. H&E stain.

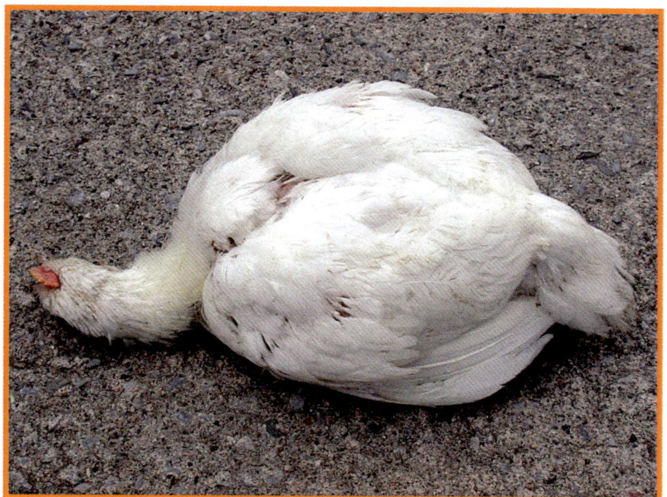

Fig. 149 | Bird with transient flaccid paralysis of the neck due to Marek's disease infection virus.

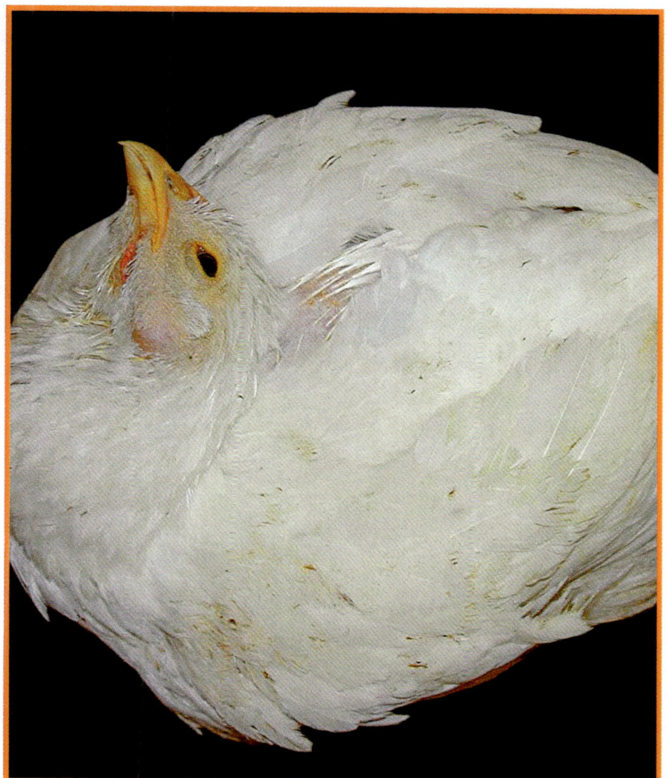

Fig. 150 | A bird with opisthotonos due to bacterial otitis and osteomyelitis.

*Ornithobacterium rhinotracheale* o *Staphylococcus hyicus*). In the latter case, the animals usually suffer from opisthotonos or torticollis (fig. 150) and a gross examination identifies fibrin or caseous material in the bones surrounding the inner ear and on the brain (fig. 151).

- **Fungi:** Just like bacterial infections, fungal infections are also uncommon, and include the formation of granulomas in the brain granulomatous encephalitis. They may be secondary to fungal pulmonary infections (*Aspergillus* spp.) or primary (*Ochroconis gallopavum*). Granulomatous encephalitis may also be seen in *Mycobacterium avium* infections.

## Peripheral Nervous System

Although other nerves may be examined, the usual one to evaluate is the sciatic nerve. The main gross lesions are enlargement of the nerves (fig. 152) and loss of striation due to Marek's disease. Affected birds suffer paralysis of the legs and lameness (fig. 153) and microscopic examination reveals neoplastic lesions, lymphomas, with intense and diffuse tumoral lymphoid cell infiltration (fig. 154). It should be remembered that lymphoproliferative disease in turkeys, or

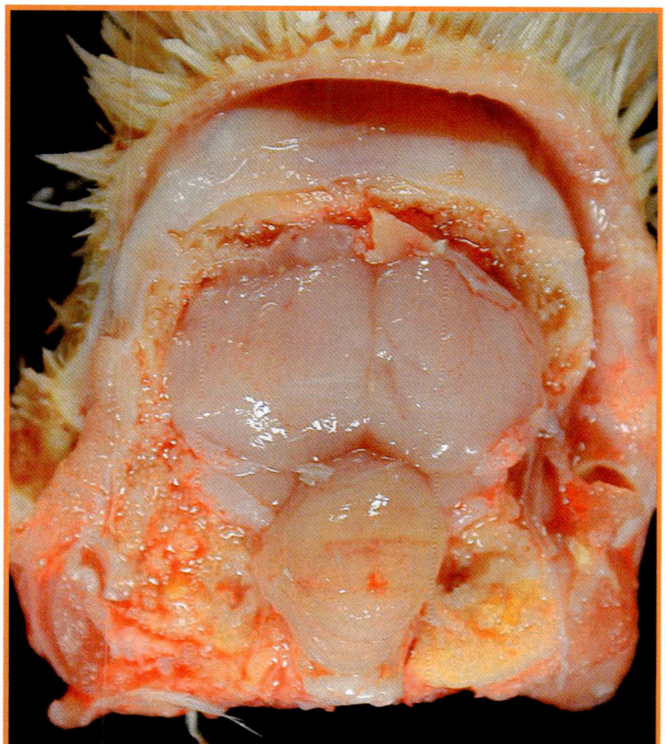

Fig. 151 | Internal otitis, osteomyelitis and granulomatous encephalitis caused by a bacterial infection of the inner ear that extends to the cerebellum. The presence of yellowish material (fibrin and necrotic material) in the bone surrounding the inner ear proves there is an inflammation.

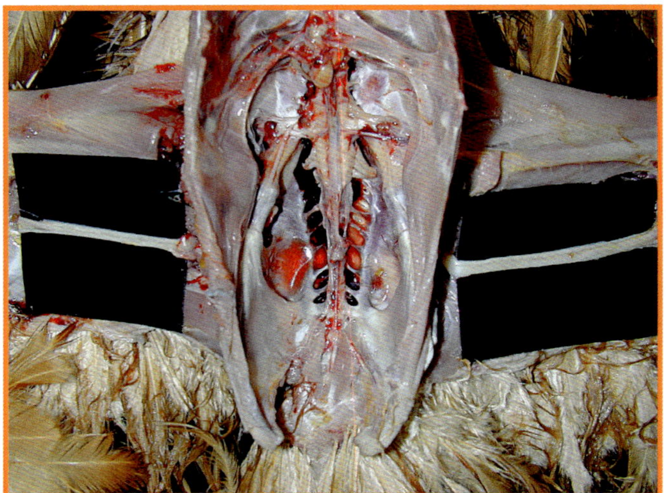
Fig. 152 | Right side sciatic nerve lymphoma in a bird affected by Marek's disease.

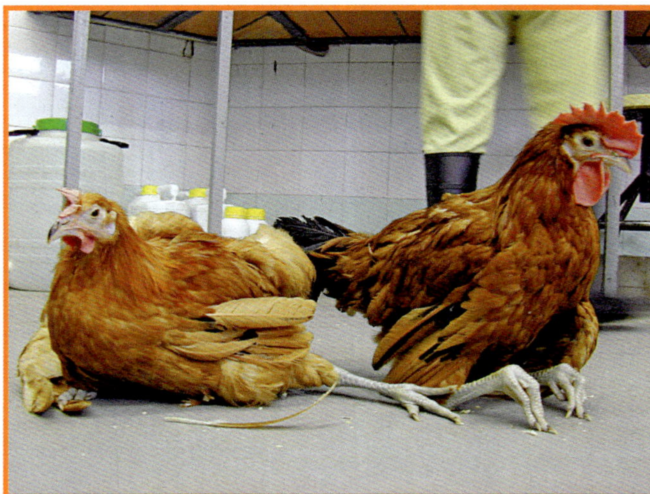
Fig. 153 | Unilateral paralysis of the leg and wing in two animals affected by Marek's disease.

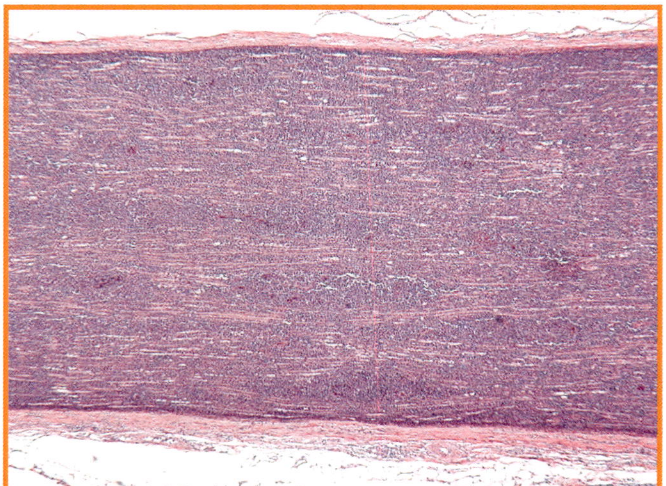
Fig. 154 | Microscopic image of a sciatic nerve lymphoma due to Marek's disease viral infection. H&E stain.

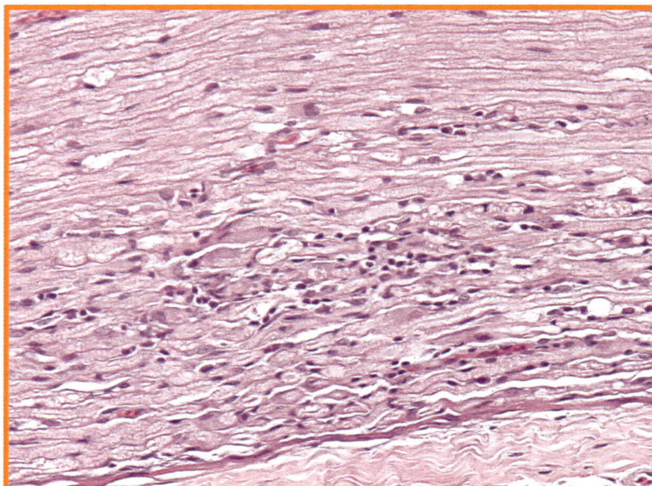
Fig. 155 | Neuritis with inflammatory focal lymphoplasmacytic infiltrate and Wallerian degeneration of axons. H&E stain.

reticuloendotheliosis in turkeys and chickens, both caused by retroviruses, may also include lymphomas in the peripheral nerves.

Although no lesions may be seen macroscopically, the absence of microscopic lesions must not be dismissed. Therefore, in some cases, usually in animals that have developed chronic Marek's disease, oedema and separation of nerve fibres, demyelination and Wallerian degeneration, together with mononuclear inflammatory infiltrate are also found (fig. 155). In the absence of tumours in other tissues, this type of lesion may also be compatible with peripheral neuropathy syndrome. This syndrome is found in 6 to 11-week-old lightweight breeder chicks, with symptoms similar to Marek's disease. Although the origin is unclear, recent studies point towards an immune-mediated disorder. Furthermore, this type of lesion is also seen in riboflavin deficiency, although in this case it affects animals less than 3 weeks of age.

CHAPTER 3

# SAMPLING AND OTHER GENERAL CONSIDERATIONS

# Practical aspects to keep in mind

As discussed in Chapter 1, a second objective of a necropsy is sampling, either to complement a diagnosis by laboratory confirmation, or for routine vaccination control, prevalence estimation, etc.

It is necessary to perform adequate sampling for the laboratory results to be valid and this requires forethought in the following areas:

- **The tissue or organ** selected for sampling. It should be selected because it will provide representative information. In some cases, this will be the tissue that has gross lesions, but in other cases it will be that which might present characteristic lesions according to the existing bibliography.
- **The type of sample** to be taken. Once the tissue or organ for the sample has been decided, the type of sample to be collected will have to be considered, which could be a portion of the organ, a plate or a FTA© plate (Flinders Technology Associates, Whatman).
- **Preservation method.** Finally, once the sample is obtained, the preservation method to be used until its arrival at the laboratory must be decided upon (e. g., submerged in formalin, cooled in refrigeration, frozen or at room temperature).

These three aspects will depend upon:

- **The laboratory study** to be performed. The type of analysis required will dictate, in large measure, the type of sample and the preservation method. Also, the pathology to be confirmed or dismissed will also affect the laboratory study.
- **The suspected pathology.** It is essential to know basic aspects about the pathology to be confirmed or dismissed, e.g. the organs which are most affected, any pathognomonic lesions in those organs, or the length of time the pathogen is detectable, in the case of an infectious process. All this information will determine which laboratory study is most adequate, and, in turn, the most appropriate samples required.

It is worth remembering that the laboratory will help with any questions or doubts, and will advise on the most pertinent laboratory study or the tests available for each pathology.

## Submitting samples to the laboratory

It should be noted that the laboratory receiving the samples does not possess as much information about the case as the veterinarian, therefore it is recommended to do the following:

1. Submit an 'analysis request form' with the samples. This should include a list of the references or samples submitted and the case history (including the type of bird, age, vaccinations, geographical area, clinical signs observed and the lesions observed at necropsy). Include the contact person's details (phone and email).
2. Correctly label the sample containers with the identification of the farm/premises or the specified reference in the case history.
3. Externally identify the package with the sender's details and the receiving laboratory's address.
4. Send the samples by courier. Above all, take into account the weekends and holidays in other postal areas, to ensure the samples are not more than 24 hours in transit.

In any case, it is recommended to give prior notice to the laboratory receiving the samples, especially if they are perishable or urgent.

# Histopathology

Histopathological studies are extremely useful tools:

1. To confirm the cause of a disease or pathology which has produced characteristic microscopic lesions. For example, the presence of intranuclear inclusion bodies and syncytial cells in the tracheal epithelium is characteristic of infectious laryngotracheitis.
2. To link the presence of an infectious agent to the existence of associated lesions. The presence of an agent does not always confirm that it is the cause of the problematic condition. For example, when molecular tests detect the presence of the Gumboro virus, it is not always associated to the IBD clinicopathological condition; it may be a vaccine strain that has been detected.
3. To guide pathological processes which have difficult clinical characterisation.

## Type of sample

The samples required for this type of study are organ or tissue portions. The tissue portion should be more or less square and measuring between 0.5 and 1 cm per side. The brain is never removed from the skull, but is fixed as a whole.

## Tissues or organs for sampling

Samples are taken from organs with lesions or organs where characteristic lesions are known to occur.

## Sample preservation

The tissues are to be fixed by immersion in diluted 10% buffered formalin (compared to the commercial form), and within plastic containers with airtight seals (fig. 1). It should be remembered that formalin in commercial form has a maximum concentration of 40%, therefore, when diluted 10 times the correct final concentration is 4%. A tissue to formalin volume ratio of 1:10 is important to achieve a proper fixation of the sample (fig. 2).

**PATHOLOGIES OF CHOICE FOR A HISTOPATHOLOGICAL STUDY**

- Marek's disease/avian leukosis.
- Adenovirus infection.
- Tuberculosis.
- Infectious laryngotracheitis/avian pox.
- Encephalomyelitis/encephalomalacia.
- Aspergillosis.
- Nutritional deficiencies.
- Parasitosis (coccidiosis).
- Tenosynovitis virus.
- Toxic or nutritional myopathies.

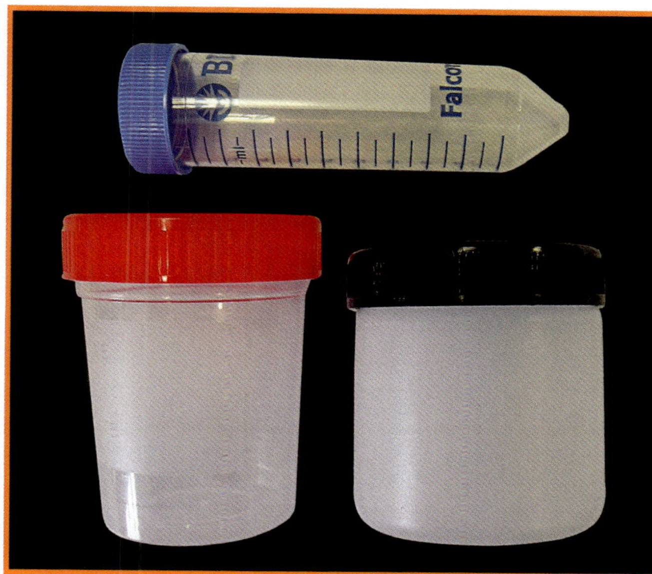

Fig. 1 | Examples of plastic containers with airtight seals.

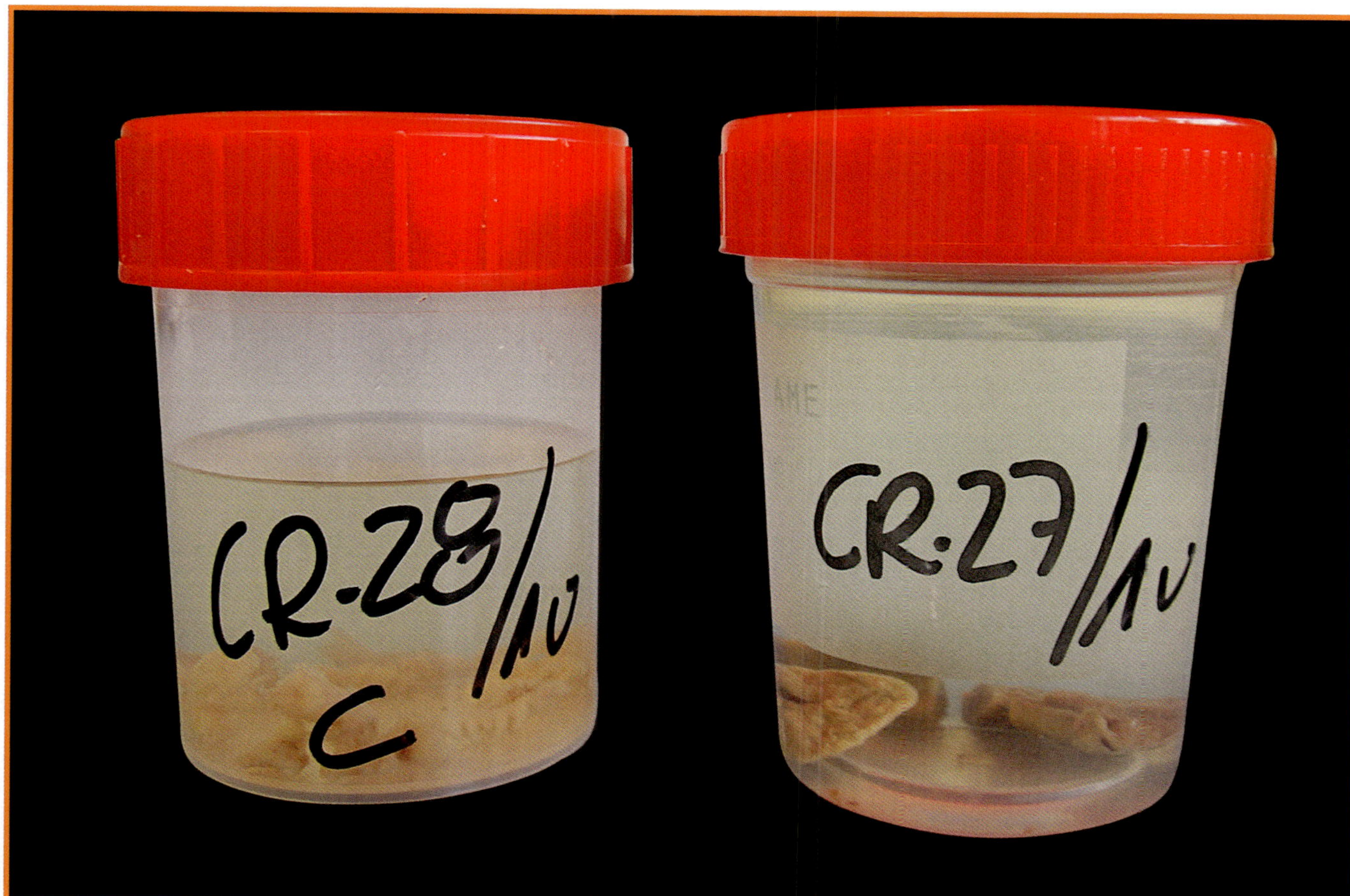


Fig. 2 | To correctly fix the sample, the ratio between the volume of tissue and the formalin should be 1:10.

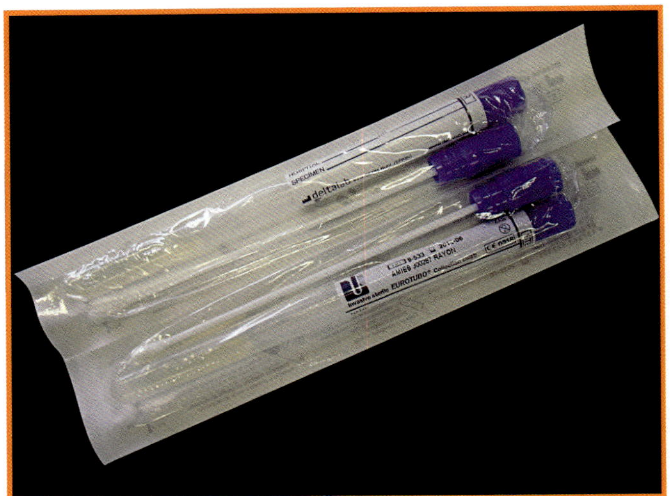


Fig. 3 | Tubes for collecting samples using swabs with transport medium.

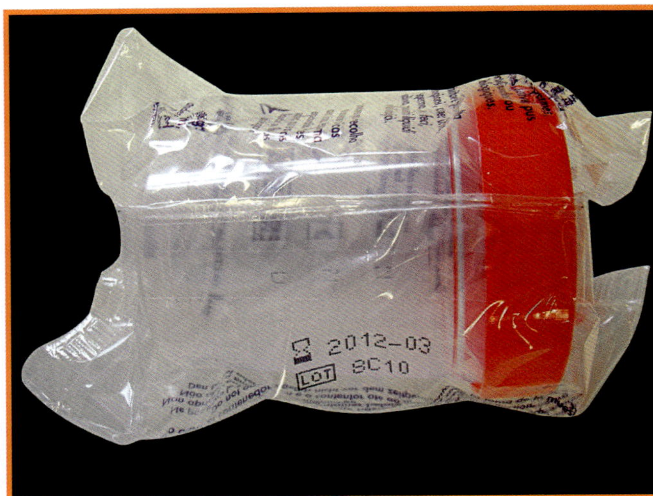


Fig. 4 | Sterile container for collecting portions of organs.

# Microbiology/bacteriology

Bacteriological studies are extremely useful tools:

1. To isolate the bacterial or fungal causative agent from the clinical profile.
2. To perform an antibiogram, which helps to identify the potentially more efficient antibiotic treatment.

## Type of sample

Microbiological study samples may be collected using a swab, preferably with transport medium (fig. 3) or by extracting a portion of an organ which is introduced into a sterile flask in the maximum sterile conditions possible (fig. 4).

## Tissues or organs for sampling

- Generally, the organ or tissue of choice is the one where macroscopic lesions indicative of bacterial infection are observed.
- In cases where septicaemia is suspected, even though lesions are not observable, it is advisable to sample at least two or three tissues from each bird, in order to confirm the presence of bacteria in various tissues.
- In the case of intestinal bacteria or intestinal bacterial counts, the sample of choice is the intestinal content from the section in which the count should take place. One option for intestinal sampling in maximum sterility is to perform a ligature at both ends of the segment of interest, and cut before the ligature at the beginning of the segment and after the ligature at the end.

In any case, the veterinarian should guide the laboratory on the suspect microbiological agents, so that the laboratory uses the most appropriate means to isolate them. For example, a specific request should be made to detect *Salmonella*, as it is a bacterium which requires a specific culture medium for its isolation.

## Sample preservation

Since some bacteria do not hold up well to freezing, it is best to keep these samples refrigerated. When taking swabs, the use of general transport medium is recommended as it retains bacterial viability for later identification.

## Pathologies of choice

In all bacterial or fungal aetiologies in which the microorganism is easily isolated.

# Virology

The objective of virological studies is to isolate the virus. In contrast to most bacteria or fungi, virus isolation is costly both in time and expense; many passes are often required to isolate the virus. Therefore, few laboratories perform this study as a routine test. These negative aspects have led to the development of molecular diagnostic techniques in recent years, which allow viruses to be detected more rapidly.

Despite this, in cases where serotype or protectotype studies are required, virus isolation is still necessary.

## Type of sample

As in bacteriological studies, the collection of samples for virus isolation can be performed from a swab or a tissue sample.

## Tissues or organs for sampling

Samples will be taken from tissues where the virus replicates, which generally coincide with the tissues in which the lesions appear. In the case of intestinal viruses, isolation can be performed from the faeces or intestinal contents.

## Sample preservation

Freezing is the best way to preserve viral viability. However, in some cases, standard freezing at -20°C is not enough. For this reason, it is best to submit samples refrigerated and by courier.

**PATHOLOGIES OF CHOICE FOR A VIROLOGICAL STUDY**

- Avian infectious bronchitis.
- Avian infectious laryngotracheitis.
- Avian pox.
- Adenovirus infection.
- Avian influenza.
- Newcastle disease.

# Molecular biology

Molecular studies are extremely useful tools:

1. To detect bacterial, viral or parasitic pathogens, such as *Mycoplasma synoviae*, which in general are costly to isolate.
2. To genotype the pathogens. In many cases the molecular tests allow the causative agent to not only be detected but also to be characterised better: by distinguishing different types of strains or distinguishing between field strains and vaccine strains. As mentioned earlier, the molecular characterisation of the Gumboro virus detects and differentiates the strain of the vaccine virus from the field strain.
3. Quantification of pathogens. Some techniques determine the exact copy number of genomes present in a sample. Although currently these techniques are mostly used on an experimental level, in the future they might be useful in diagnosing certain pathologies.

## Type of sample

The collection of samples for molecular studies is obtained by a swab or a portion of tissue. It should be remembered, that in this study the swabs must be dry, without any transport media (fig. 5). Also it may be useful to obtain FTA-card spots in some pathogens (for example, in the case of Gumboro virus). It has been demonstrated that these cards inactivate the infectious agent but preserve its genetic material, and therfore may be used in these techniques. However, it must be remembered that it is not possible to isolate the microorganism from these cards at a later date.

## Tissues or organs for sampling

The decision whether to use tissue with pathogen replication or stationary pathogen tissue will depend upon each pathogen.

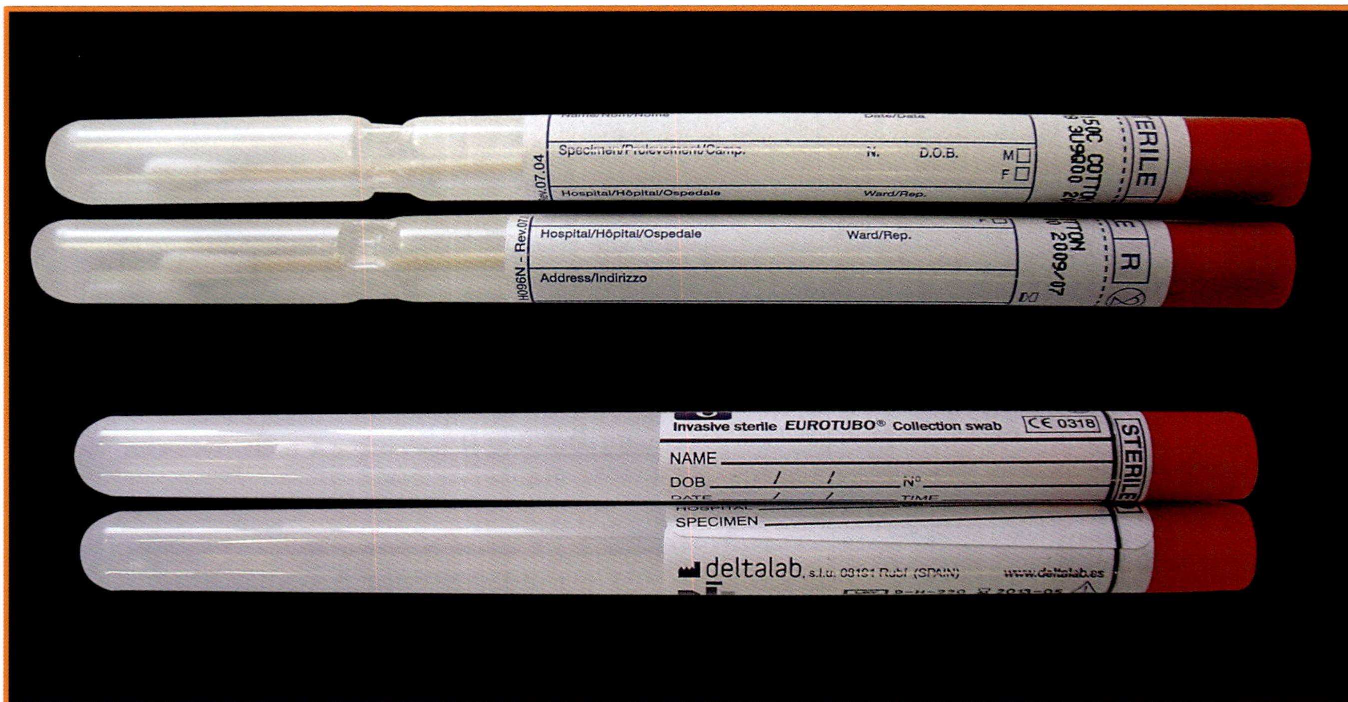


Fig. 5 | Tubes for collecting samples using swabs without transport medium.

## Sample preservation

As in virological studies, it is best to submit the samples refrigerated and by courier. Finally, the FTA-cards may be sent by regular mail at room temperature.

### PATHOLOGIES OF CHOICE FOR A MOLECULAR STUDY

- Mycoplasma.
- Avian infectious bronchitis.
- Gumboro disease.
- Avian pneumovirosis.
- Avian infectious laryngotracheitis.
- Avian influenza.
- Newcastle disease.
- Clostridium.
- Infectious coryza.
- Egg drop syndrome.

# Serology

Serology includes a set of laboratory assays to determine the presence and, in some cases, quantify the levels of antibodies compared to a particular infectious agent. Probably the most used are the ELISA and the Hemagglutination Inhibition (HAI) tests, but Rapid Plate Agglutination (RPA) or Virus Neutralisation (VN) are also performed.

Serological techniques are particularly useful tools:

- In chronic clinical profiles. When the symptoms are older than two weeks, and for that reason detecting the infectious agent is more unlikely.
- In those pathologies in which there are no existing tests to directly detect the infectious agent.
- To monitor vaccine responses.

## Type of sample

In all cases the sample is blood. As discussed in Chapter 1, the most common location to extract blood from a bird is from the basilic vein (wing vein). In the case of very young birds, the jugular would be the vein of choice.

## Sample preservation

For birds, polypropylene plastic tubes (rather than glass or other plastic tubes) are recommended as they facilitate the separation of the serum from other blood components (fig. 6). The tubes must be without anticoagulant, as the objective is for the blood to clot. In addition, other aspects should be taken into account, such as the following:

1. The tube should never be filled entirely, unless special serum separator tubes are being used, which contain gel or plastic particles.
2. After obtaining the blood, place the tube horizontally to increase the clotting surface.
3. If the samples are sent by courier they are to be sent at room temperature. If they should be preserved before being sent to the laboratory, it is advisable to maintain the temperature at 4°C.
4. Do not freeze under any conditions.
5. The serum should be separated from the clot as soon as possible to avoid haemolysis. Therefore, if it will be more than two days before the samples are sent, it is best to separate the serum into new tubes.

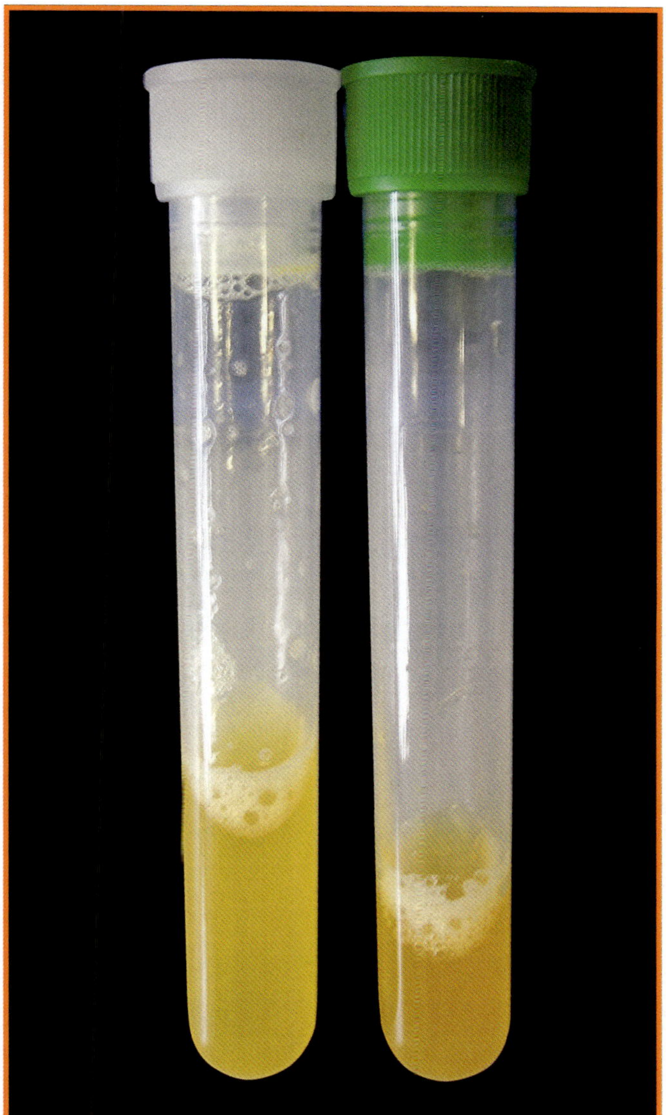

Fig. 6 | Appearance of two serum samples in good condition.

## Sample size

Serological tests are relatively inexpensive and they allow for a large number of samples to be analysed. Moreover, to obtain a meaningful result it is necessary to have a representative number of samples, thus, the larger the batch, the greater the number of samples that should be taken. Practically, it is recommended to use a minimum of 20 samples in batches of broilers and 30 in batches of breeders or layers. Never should fewer than 10 samples be taken.

### Time of sampling

It should be noted that the antibodies appear after being infected by the pathogen and that, approximately, the first antibodies at a systemic level will be found one week post infection. This means that if the seroconversion is more or less complete, then birds should be sampled two weeks after observing the clinical signs or after vaccination. If the tests are to demonstrate seroconversion, then sampling should be done at the onset of the clinical condition and 2-3 weeks later.

### Interpretation of results

Especially in regards to the ELISA tests there are a variety of commercial kits available for the same disease, which may present differences in sensitivity and specificity. For this reason, it is advisable not to directly compare results from different kits.

**PATHOLOGIES OF CHOICE FOR A SEROLOGICAL STUDY**

- Gumboro disease.
- Avian infectious bronchitis.
- Avian infectious laryngotracheitis.
- Mycoplasma.
- Avian infectious anaemia.
- Avian pneumovirosis.
- Newcastle disease.

## Parasitology

Parasitological studies are extremely useful tools:

1. To classify parasites.
2. For routine oocyst counts to monitor coccidiosis.

### Type of sample

In cases of oocyst counts, the preferred samples are mixtures (*pools*) of faeces. In the case of sampling ectoparasites or endoparasites to determine the class or species, the sample of choice would be the parasites themselves.

### Sample preservation

The faeces can be stored at room temperature due to the high resistance of oocysts. In the case of transferring parasites for classification, they should be kept in ethanol at 96%.

## Toxicology

Toxicological studies are extremely useful tools:

1. To detect the level of external toxins.
2. To determine the presence of biological toxins such as botulinum toxin or mycotoxins.

The main drawback of toxicological studies is that the veterinarian must decide which toxin to test for. There are toxins that cause specific gross or microscopic lesions, such as oosporein in the kidney, but the associated lesions in most toxins are very nonspecific or even non-existent and this makes the diagnostic very difficult to assess. Moreover, tests do not exist to identify every specific toxin, and the tests that do exist are only available in specialised laboratories (not as routine tests). Therefore, generally, the tests are not used for routine clinical diagnosis.

### Type of sample

The sample of choice for detecting external toxins or mycotoxins is the one in which the toxin is suspected to be present (e.g. water, feed, litter, etc.). To detect the botulinum toxin, the sample of choice is the serum of the affected birds.

### Sample preservation

The preservation of the sample depends upon the nature of the sample. For example, samples of feed or litter may be stored at room temperature while samples of tissue or organs, including serum, should be frozen.

Published by Servet editorial - Grupo Asís Biomedia S.L.